BEYOND CARING

MORALITY AND SOCIETY
A SERIES EDITED BY ALAN WOLFE

DANIEL F. CHAMBLISS

Beyond Caring

Hospitals, Nurses, and the
Social Organization of Ethics

THE UNIVERSITY OF CHICAGO PRESS

Chicago & London

The University of Chicago Press, Chicago 60637
The University of Chicago Press, Ltd., London
© 1996 by The University of Chicago
All rights reserved. Published 1996
Printed in the United States of America
05 04 03 02 01 00 99 98 97   2 3 4 5

ISBN 0-226-10071-5 (cloth)
0-226-10102-9 (paper)

Library of Congress Cataloging-in-Publication Data

Chambliss, Daniel F.
    Beyond caring : hospitals, nurses, and the social organization of
ethics / Daniel F. Chambliss.
        p.   cm. — (Morality and society)
    Includes bibliographical references and index.
    1. Nursing ethics.   2. Hospital care—Moral and ethical aspects.
3. Nurses—Job stress.   4. Role conflict.   5. Nurses—Attitudes.
I. Title.   II. Series.
RT85.C48   1996
174'.2—dc20   95-42835
                                                     CIP

This book is dedicated to my mother,

to the memory of my father,

and to my confidant, ping-pong buddy,

and friend for life, David Collins.

CONTENTS

Acknowledgments

This project has spanned nearly fifteen years and has been influenced by countless people: research subjects, academic colleagues, friends, and advisors. Only a comparative handful of these people can be named here, but I want the others to know that I appreciate their help and, if anything, am sorry that I haven't made better use of their contributions.

First, over a hundred working nurses allowed me to interview them formally, and many more permitted me to watch them at work, listen in on their conversations, and ask them all sorts of questions. In addition, administrators, physicians, and affiliated hospital staff people were helpful as well in a variety of ways. I promised all these people confidentiality at the time, and I thank them now as a group. Their support and openness were crucial.

Kai Erikson guided the earliest phase of the project as my Ph.D. dissertation advisor at Yale. His professional encouragement and personal friendship over the past fifteen years have been invaluable. Rosabeth Kanter, Maurice Natanson, and Raymond Duff, M.D., in various ways shaped my thinking and were wonderful graduate teachers.

Since I left Yale in 1981, my "teachers" have been colleagues and friends whose intellectual abilities I admire and hope in some small ways to emulate: Lynn Chancer, Randall Collins, Dan Ryan, and Eviatar Zerubavel have been such teachers; and Alfred Kelly has contributed in countless ways, too many to mention, over the past fourteen years. At Hamilton, my senior colleagues in sociology, David Gray and Dennis Gilbert, have been wonderfully supportive from the beginning. ix

Indeed, I believe that Hamilton College as an institution, in particular under the leadership of Dean and now President Eugene Tobin, is unequaled in its support of professionally active teaching scholars. Howard S. Becker, Alan Wolfe, and Robert Zussman, as manuscript reviewers for the University of Chicago Press, made detailed comments as well as strategic suggestions that I have tried to incorporate. And three registered nurses who have been good friends for years provided detailed comments on drafts and answered innumerable questions, and I am deeply grateful to them: Patricia Galloway, Joan Greening, and Deborah Southwick.

Financial support came from several sources. Throughout the project Hamilton College has been wonderfully generous, providing paid leaves through Margaret Bundy Scott Fellowships as well as travel and research funds. A Rockefeller Foundation Fellowship at the Institute for the Medical Humanities, University of Texas Medical Branch, provided time for drafting the main plan for the book and testing my theories against the collected wisdom of a talented and diverse faculty of humanists. Professor Ronald Carson, director of the institute, and his colleagues were always helpful and frequently inspiring. A Fulbright lectureship to the University of Iceland gave me time in a peaceful setting to rework some of the material and visit with nurses in a totally different health care system.

Student research assistants at Hamilton tracked down references, copied articles, reorganized files, kept me on schedule, and carried out a wide array of miscellaneous tasks with enthusiasm: Christina Cosgrove Cawley, Jody Speier Dietz, Bill Russell, and Nina Schmergel.

Ever since we first met in 1981, Doug Mitchell of the University of Chicago Press has been encouraging and intelligently critical of this project and others; I always wanted this Press and this editor for this book, and I am happy with that choice.

Laurie Moses and Theresa George typed the dissertation manuscript and helped in numerous ways in the earliest stages of the work.

Janice Pieroni, a first-rate professional secretary, after years of typing drafts and correcting my sometimes bizarre writing errors, prepared the entire manuscript to exacting specifications. In countless ways over the past eight years she has held my work to her own high standards. I am deeply grateful.

Finally, two friends deserve special notice. Penny Rosel, my undergraduate advisor at New College, not only started me in sociology but, more importantly, has been an extraordinary model for how one should live as a teacher and a human being. And Lawton Harper, a former student who is now in every sense a friend and colleague, really made the completion of this book possible: not least, by calling at 6:30 A.M. every morning to check if I was up and working on it. Of such mundane events are books made—and wonderful friendships as well.

Nursing and Ethics
in an Age of Organizations

Nursing is a noble profession but too often a terrible job. At its best, nursing is a calling, a physically and emotionally challenging, humanly fulfilling moral mission. Nurses encounter patients in their most vulnerable moments, sharing an intimacy found in few other human relationships. Sometimes they work with a personal commitment transcending technical performance, a commitment too rarely found in most careers. At the same time, nurses express frustration as their immediate, even dominant, emotional response to their work. "I can't do my job," they say. "There is no support from the higher ups." Lack of time, of support, of supplies, of respect are mentioned again and again. In letters to nursing magazines, the theme is echoed: "I love nursing, *but* . . ." There is, in many nurses' daily lives, the constant conflict between what nursing at its best could be—the ideal—and what too often it actually is—the reality. For many nurses, the tension is intolerable. By the late 1980s, despite historically high salaries, multithousand-dollar signing bonuses, wide-open career ladders, despite work that produces immediately tangible results, despite great opportunities for learning, and despite the virtual guarantee of employment for nurses who wanted to work,[1] nearly one-third of

---

1. "[H]istorically nurses have been fully employed. That is, any nurse who wants to work can find a job. Therefore, the supply of nurses [in economic terms] is considered to be the same as the population of employed registered nurses." American Nurses' Association, *Facts about Nursing 86–87* (Kansas City, MO: American Nurses' Association, 1987), p. 1. The total number of nurses in practice increased, between 1978 and 1985, by an average of about 50,000 a year, again according to the ANA *Facts*, p. 3.

the registered nurses in the United States were not practicing nursing.

Working nurses often feel actively thwarted in their jobs, blocked from doing the meaningful work that was promised them. They feel that their professional birthright has been violated by administrators, by physicians, sometimes by government policies. Perhaps these nurses entered the profession with naive expectations. This younger generation, fresh from collegiate programs with broad classroom experience but little clinical experience, and imbued with an aggressive, independent theory of what nursing could be, comes into the hospital eager to serve, only to suffer the "reality shock" of limited resources, shortstaffing in the hospitals, and recalcitrant, chronic, incurable patients, who are not at all grateful or appreciative of the young nurse's care.[2] Perhaps nurses suffer from the inherent contradiction, as Susan Reverby puts it, of being "ordered to care":[3] *required* by one's job to do emotion work[4] which needs to be felt spontaneously. Or perhaps they are feeling the clash as a clearly female (97 percent of all nurses are women) culture of personal relationships meets with the impersonality of a more traditionally male organizational world.[5] And while women are rapidly entering the ranks of medical doctors, no comparable change is occurring in nursing. Whatever its source, the frustration and disappointment of many nurses is quite real, and it is often perceived in distinctly moral terms. One cannot be an ethical nurse, it may seem, in this setting where powerful others block what nurses see as their professional obligations.[6] Studying nurses' frustra-

2. See Marlene Kramer, *Reality Shock: Why Nurses Leave Nursing* (St. Louis: C. V. Mosby, 1974).

3. Susan Reverby, *Ordered to Care: The Dilemma of American Nursing, 1850–1945* (Cambridge: Cambridge University Press, 1987).

4. On the concept of "emotion work," see Arlie Russell Hochschild, *The Managed Heart* (Berkeley: University of California Press, 1983).

5. This refers to nurses who work in hospitals. "A result of the large increase in the number of nurses in hospitals between 1977 and 1984 was that hospitals employed an increasing percentage of the total supply [of nurses]. The percentage increased from 61.4 percent in 1977 to 65.7 percent in 1980, and to more than 68 percent in 1984." *Facts about Nursing*, p. 98.

6. "Thus, the hospital nurse finds herself constrained in various and occasionally conflicting ways by the hospital (which employs her), the physician (with

tions, we can learn lessons about the psychology of workers in any organization, and about the very possibility for being a moral individual in an organizational world of contending and sometimes divergent interests.

Like most working Americans, the hospital nurse is fundamentally an organization member; this profoundly affects nursing's moral position. Nurses are subordinated to hospital authority in numerous ways, subject to its policies, directed by its head nurses, its supervisors, and its administrators. They are subordinate as well to the orders of numerous physicians and must work within doctors' vision of the patient's needs and their plans for the patient's life, or death. But in this dual subordination to the hospital's bureaucracy and the physician's orders, nurses may forget their profession's distinctive goals. As nurses tell it, nursing's moral core, its commitment to the welfare of the patient as a "whole person," has been buried under medical directives and the financial and administrative imperatives of the modern medical center. In a setting where one's work is governed by others, how can one person claim her own moral integrity? Perhaps with the decline of nursing orders of religious nuns, the spiritual commitment that many nurses once felt has been replaced by a more secular, instrumentalist view of their profession. And perhaps, too, nursing is hidden behind medicine: witness the great prestige of the highly technological methods of the Intensive Care Unit, the mechanical heart and lung, the artificial kidneys of Dialysis Units, and the mystique and financial power of medical research, in which as much as $1,000,000 is spent on a single interesting case,[7] while dozens of old people throughout the hospital lie in bed waiting for lunch. Nurses complain of this and say, in their own words, that nursing has lost its own moral footing.

---

whom she works), the client (for whom she provides care), and the nursing profession (to which she belongs). To what extent can she be her own person—i.e., be ethically autonomous—in these circumstances?" Martin Benjamin and Joy Curtis, *Ethics in Nursing* (New York: Oxford University Press, 1981), p. 23.

7. "Case," not "patient," is the correct word here. The money is spent not because the patient is a valuable person but because his or her malady is of interest to medical researchers. The patient, we might say, is the setting for the experiment.

My topic here, then, is somewhat broader than "ethics" as usually conceived. Morality is the more general term, applying to human experiences of right and wrong in everyday life. Moral issues are often unformulated, even unconscious; morality can even refer to the general *tone* of a world. Ethics, on the other hand, refers to a more conscious reflection on our moral beliefs, and seems typically to be applied to specific cases in a setting as opposed to the nature of the setting itself. In professional settings such as hospitals, "ethics" usually refers to the codification of moral principles by an occupational group (as in "medical ethics"); often, the code reflects the group's long-range self-interest in its image as a servant of the community.

This codification of moral values can have sociological effects: it frames debate in its own terms. Once an ethical vocabulary is adopted, subsequent arguments must fit into its terminology; thus, it controls the assumptions of debate. In medicine, the use of bioethical language has made moral debates more abstract (by continually referring to general principles), rights-driven, individualistic, and centered on discrete cases. Left aside, often, are discussions of the general routines or structures of medical services. Such language is legalistic in tone and sometimes indistinguishable from legal advice. An "ethics consultation" in American hospitals often includes the hospital lawyer, and decisions on what is right are regularly tempered by what the courts officially sanction as legal. Where the language of ethics frames debate, certain issues find no place in the conversation. At the same time, this language can be a weapon for those who know it: for nurses, the revolution of bioethics has provided words, phrases, and arguments to use in their conflicts with physicians and administrators.

Still, this language was not created with nursing in mind, and the discipline of bioethics, recently expanded from medical ethics, has for the most part bypassed nursing.[8] Perhaps

8. The preeminent text in the field, *Principles of Biomedical Ethics*, 3d ed., by Tom L. Beauchamp and James F. Childress (New York: Oxford University Press, 1989), indexes a mention of nursing for 29 pages of its 452 pages of printed text; in a number of these instances, the word is used with little or no substantive discussion of the position of nursing specifically. Perhaps the

that is appropriate. Ethics aims to answer the question "What should be done?" Hence, in its practical applications, it is written for powerful people who make decisions, not the powerless who carry them out. Physicians are the ones who write informed consent protocols and Do Not Resuscitate orders, and perform abortions. Medical researchers suffer ethical dilemmas, choosing between the two worthy ends of knowledge and future benefits, on the one hand, and the health and comfort of the current patient on the other.[9] Doctors ask, and can decide, "How do we choose?" Ethics provides well-considered answers for them which are logically derived from clear principles.

But perhaps in speaking to powerful decision makers, traditional ethics leaves the rest of us behind. Most people don't exercise the power that physicians do. Certainly most health care workers don't. A large proportion of the American labor force works in large bureaucracies, where their work is planned to the smallest detail by absent others. Discussions of the ethics of life and death pose difficult questions, but the answers given by most people won't matter. How, a nurse may reasonably ask, should one act when one *isn't* powerful?

In other respects, too, traditional bioethics has left aside the world in which nurses, and most other people, live. In 1979, when I first began research in this field, I read a series of publications by one of the better-known clearinghouses for bioethics literature. I was quickly frustrated by the detachment of it all from what actually happens in hospitals. Ethicists would

outstanding monograph of the field, Paul Ramsey's *The Patient as Person* (New Haven: Yale University Press, 1970), has no index mention of nursing at all but is dedicated "For Jenifer Ramsey, nurse"; and a major handbook for practice, *Clinical Ethics*, by Albert R. Jonsen, Mark Siegler, and William J. Winslade (New York: Macmillan, 1982), although it has no index, does have a "Locator" which has multiple listings for "patient-physician relationship" and "physician responsibility," but has no mention whatsoever of nursing. This is not unreasonable; medical ethics is geared primarily to physicians. The point is that nursing, which will actually carry out many of the decisions, has no place in the discussion.

9. Or between the researcher's own career advancement and the welfare of the immediate patient. Physicians are aware themselves of this dilemma, and many of them honestly struggle with their own motives.

fabricate difficult, even bizarre, hypothetical case scenarios designed to test their acuity in applying one or another principle and, balancing carefully, would then develop a series of possible resolutions to the case presented. Such exercises were framed by hypothetical questions, not real situations. They were designed, I thought, not to replicate crucial features of reality but to generate the toughest test of a philosopher's logic.[10] Too often, then, it seems that in asking "What should be done?" philosophers ignore a prior question: "What *can* be done?" Much of bioethics assumes that people are autonomous decision makers sitting in a fairly comfortable room trying logically to fit problems to given solution-making patterns. The whole business is almost deliberately unreal—intellectually challenging but not very useful. And when bioethics does handle real issues, its solutions remain basically academic. Inside hospitals, by contrast, decisions are driven not by academic problem-solving techniques but by the routines of life in a professional bureaucracy. Efforts to teach powerless second-year medical students "four principles of ethics"[11] do little to alter those routines.[12]

A more empirical approach to bioethics research, focusing on nursing, could shift the debate in several ways: (1) It would move discussions from the hypothetical scenarios to real set-

10. "Questions surrounding the limitation of treatment have generated rich literatures in medical ethics, filled with fine distinctions and carefully drawn conclusions from clearly formulated principles. But medical ethics is one thing; medical practice is quite another." Robert Zussman, *Intensive Care* (Chicago: University of Chicago Press, 1992), p. 100.

11. The four proposed in Beauchamp and Childress, *Principles of Biomedical Ethics:* respect for autonomy, nonmaleficence, beneficence, and justice.

12. Near the conclusion of a detailed quantitative study of how physicians actually make ethics decisions, Diana Crane writes that "ethical codes generally specify desirable consequences of physician behavior. However, it appears that such codes are of limited usefulness. It is more important to specify the organizational variables conducive to ethical behavior." Diana Crane, *The Sanctity of Social Life: Physicians' Treatment of Critically Ill Patients* (New Brunswick: Transaction Books, 1977), p. 195. This first paperback edition, with new material, is copyrighted by the Russell Sage Foundation. More succinctly, Andrew Jameton writes, "Ideas are not solutions to ethical problems; new ways of life are." *Nursing Practice: The Ethical Issues* (Englewood Cliffs, NJ: Prentice-Hall, 1984), p. xvii.

tings. We understand the abstract logic of ethics, but the social and psychological realities of hospital life are only just beginning to emerge. (2) It would move ethics from a formal individualism to a broader organizational awareness. Nursing's problems in particular reflect the organizational structures in which nurses work, and any serious discussion of ethics in nursing must deal with these realities. In looking at nurses' ethical difficulties, we necessarily learn about life in organizations. (3) Finally, empirical study would move ethics from speaking only of the few people who are autonomous to speaking of the many relatively powerless who work in organizations; we will have to deal with politics.[13] Nurses, being employees, deal not so much with tragic choices as with practical, often political, issues of cajoling, tricking, or badgering a recalcitrant system into doing what ought to be done. Nurses continue to admire Florence Nightingale because she did what should be done, and did so without being fired. Certainly the principles and methods of bioethics can clarify the issues and specify what choices are being faced. But sometimes clarification only makes obvious the opposed goals of the battling factions. And if that is so, then a seminar on "great issues in bioethics" won't help much; lectures by prominent speakers miss the point; changing an individual's consciousness, one individual at a time, won't solve any problems. In fact, such efforts at ameliorating ethical lapses may well be a distraction, fostering a public impression that something is being done. The real problems then go untouched and remain where they always were, embedded in organizational routines and structures.

Political considerations touch directly onto questions of ethics. For instance, frequently arguments arise within the hospital regarding whether an issue is one of ethics, and hence moral debate, or of technical judgment, hence professional expertise. Ethics involves broadly human questions, answer-

---

13. And with the work of sociology: "[I]t is precisely all the processes involved in the definition and enforcement of moral rule that form the core problems of sociology." Everett C. Hughes, "Mistakes at Work," in *Men and Their Work* (Westport, CT: Greenwood Press, [1958] 1981), p. 101. Jameton's *Nursing Practice* is remarkable for the way in which it does speak directly to the practicalities of organizational life. But then, as a book about nursing, not medicine, it needs to.

able outside the confines of any particular discipline or specialty.[14] While nurses may recognize a technique (say, the insertion of chest tubes for drainage) as being in the physician's sphere of competence, the corresponding ethical question (whether chest tubes should be placed in a hopelessly ill patient) may be regarded as answerable more or less by any sensible human being. For the moral decision, technical training is irrelevant.

In questions of sustaining life, a physician may claim that, based on long training and an understanding of pathophysiology, he or she should decide when treatment will cease; while nurses in the same setting may contend that the question is rather one of the patient's autonomy, dignity, and the like, and that all parties involved should participate in the decision. When treatment does cease and "palliation" begins, then nurses are in charge of the case. Such an argument is less a question of ethics than of power and of who will make the decision. What officially appears as an ethics argument is actually a thinly disguised turf battle.

An empirical approach to nursing ethics in particular would also recognize the central role of gender in such arguments. Both the people and the ethos of nursing are predominantly feminine, and this shapes the problems seen and solutions practiced. By now we have good evidence that men and women frequently conceive of moral problems in somewhat different ways. In nursing, I will argue, the structural features of the work may be more important than one's gender or personal preferences for action, but even the structural requirements reinforce a "female" style. Even while avoiding any reification of the differences in masculine and feminine "moral reasoning," we can still take note of these differences and see how they play out in the hospital. Because almost all nurses are women, it is hard to separate what is "female" from what is "nursing," but we do find hints. And only an empirical study can make that distinction.

So this is a work of social science, not logical or moral philosophy. I will not begin with a philosophical definition of

14. Some writers, Jameton for one, would add that ethics refers to professional behavior, morals to personal.

"ethics" or conclude with a prescription for nurses' behavior. I am not trained in the dialectics of moral argument or in the propositions and truth tables of logic. This is sociology; my task is to describe in detail, and with defensible generalizations, how nurses define and respond to ethical problems in their daily work. I will describe the factors that shape the nurse's experience of ethical difficulties, as she herself defines them. Although the literature on nursing and health care has been used here[15], the findings rest primarily on my own fieldwork. The research has been empirical; the data are mostly events I have seen myself or have been told of by participants.[16]

The research was conducted between 1979 and 1990, in three discrete blocks: the first, from January 1979 until June 1980, in a large Northeastern medical center; the second, from June through August of 1982, in a mid-sized (300-bed) community hospital also in the Northeast; and the third, from January until June of 1990, in a large medical center in the Southwest. I also spent short periods in other hospitals, both in America and abroad. This totals over two years of full-time work, including some 110 formal interviews and countless days and nights of on-site observation of nurses at work.[17] The research was thus extensive, covering a long period of time, across the geography of the United States, in many different units of a number of hospitals, and with a sizable number of nurses. During this eleven-year period, ethics committees became common in hospitals, the federal government began monitoring life-support decisions (in the "Baby Doe" regulations), Do Not Resuscitate policies became mandatory, and the spreading impact of the women's movement came to be felt throughout the workplace. All of these changes were evident over the course of the research. Things were not in 1990 as they had been in 1979.

This book looks at the experience of nurses and how they

15. Diana Crane's *The Sanctity of Social Life* is an early example of a sociological/empirical approach to medical ethics; so is Charles L. Bosk, *Forgive and Remember: Managing Medical Failure* (Chicago: University of Chicago Press, 1979).
16. Citations to other authors are given in footnotes.
17. See the Appendix on Methods, this volume.

live their moral lives. We will see that their moral feelings and daily actions are not separate entities and that a host of moral assumptions are embedded in their habitual modes of behavior.[18] The individual nurse and her setting are integrally joined; indeed, the individual and her setting are reciprocally, mutually defining. A nurse is truly a nurse only if she has patients;[19] similarly, a hospital nurse is irredeemably a part of the hospital of which she is a part. Neither the hospital nor the nurse can entirely distinguish itself from the other. In this context, we see how the nurse's self and role are intertwined with her experience of the hospital, her patients, and her work. There may be, as we will see in Chapter Six, an effort to detach herself from the work she does; but these efforts are typically characterized by their continuing, relapsing failure. Simply, we will explore the moral geography of hospital nursing. In a broader sense we will be detailing what it means, in experiential terms, to be a member of an organization.[20]

The argument is developed through six chapters and a Conclusion. In Chapters One and Two, we will see how the terrible reality of the hospital, so abnormal for most of us, becomes transformed into a routine; and then how that routine is protected when emergencies arise. Ethical issues exist not as freestanding problems but, instead, as embedded in complexes of routine and emergency, often very different from those seen by outsiders to the organization. With this different background, the ethical problems of nurses are different. In Chapter Three, I will try to explain what it means to "be a nurse" in the hospital; we will look at the nurse's role and how it includes her subordination to the goals and plans

18. For an exposition, in the case of expert nurses, of what that embedded knowledge actually includes, see Patricia Benner, *From Novice to Expert: Excellence and Power in Clinical Nursing Practice* (Menlo Park, CA: Addison-Wesley, 1984).

19. Certainly many nurse administrators identify themselves as nurses, despite their distance from the bedside. My point is that identity as a nurse implies a relationship to patients, just as one cannot be a mother without having had a child.

20. This approach derives from phenomenological philosophy as applied to social science, especially the works of Alfred Schutz, Jean-Paul Sartre, Maurice Merleau-Ponty, and Maurice Natanson.

of others. In Chapter Four, we will show how the hospital itself is not a neutral setting but is actually the creator of many of the nurse's ethical difficulties. Ethical difficulties are not indicative of unintended flaws in the system but are instead expressions of that system in its most basic features. In particular, ethical problems are an expression of interest group conflict played out in the hospital.[21] If this is correct, then individualistic solutions to ethical issues can never provide lasting solutions. Chapter Five looks at how hospitals turn patients into relatively passive recipients of biomedical treatment, into *objects*. This transformation, made possible by the power of the medical staffs to impose their view of disease, leads to many of the ethical problems nurses encounter. Despite hospital actions, patients reject such treatment, creating ethical problems for the staff. Chapter Six describes one common response nurses make to ethical problems: the detachment of the self from its own behavior. In cases where nurses bring pain or death to patients, nurses often psychologically separate themselves from what they are doing, denying that "I" was really involved at all. This is a delimitation of responsibility, a marking off of the limits of one's own accountability for the world. This sort of alienation from work is a common feature of organizational life. Finally, the Conclusion will address the relevance of this study to ethics, nursing, and sociology, and close with a few hopeful comments for the future.

All of this may teach us about the morality of medical settings in which, in the most helpless moments of our lives, we must truly rely upon the kindness of strangers.

21. Indeed, the field of medical ethics itself can be seen as a player in these battles: "The starting point, then, for any sociology of medical ethics must be a recognition that the very field itself is both symptom and, to some degree, cause of the waning of medicine's authority." Zussman, *Intensive Care*, p. 4.

ONE

The Routinization
of Disaster

The moral system of the nurse's world, the hospital, is quite different from that of the lay world. In the hospital it is the good people, not the bad, who take knives and cut people open; here the good stick others with needles and push fingers into rectums and vaginas, tubes into urethras, needles into the scalp of a baby; here the good, doing good, peel dead skin from a screaming burn victim's body and tell strangers to take off their clothes. Here, in the words of an old joke, the healthy take money from the sick, and the most skilled cut up old ladies and get paid for it. The layperson's horrible fantasies here become the professional's stock in trade.[1] Some people believe, reasonably, that nurses' work must, therefore, be terribly stressful. "How do they cope with it?" is a question I am frequently asked. But the layperson has not seen the routinization of activities and the parallel flattening of emotion that takes place as one becomes a nurse. Nursing is stressful, to be sure, but not in the way the layperson imagines. Intravenous lines started, meds delivered, baths given, trays passed out, vital signs taken, a nonstop round of filling out forms, of writing reports, sending off blood samples—this fills the nurse's day, routine tasks done dozens of times. The moral ambiguity of any one task becomes utterly lost in the pile of repeated events; the routine blurs the moral difficulties.

1. The idea comes from Everett C. Hughes, "Mistakes at Work," reprinted in Hughes, *The Sociological Eye: Selected Papers*, with a New Introduction by David Reisman and Howard S. Becker (New Brunswick: Transaction Books, 1984), pp. 316–326.

Problems arise against this background of routine. In the large medical center, deaths occur every day. Only a few of them become "ethics problems" for the staff: a patient wants to die, and the staff won't let her; when the staff does let her die, then the family doesn't understand why. Tests and procedures cause pain, but few tests and procedures are challenged on moral grounds. Privacy is violated in the most egregious ways, all the time; but usually the violation is unhappily accepted by the suffering patient, who understands that the professional is just doing her job.

This chapter will detail how the routinization of this abnormal world occurs; Chapter Two will show how, even in the face of chaos, the routine is maintained.

THE HOSPITAL SETTING

As a formal organization, the hospital can be readily described, in objective terms, as a professional bureaucracy. For readers unfamiliar with general hospitals, a brief description of the organization, and some key terms describing its structure, will be useful.

Consider Northern General, one of the hospitals where this research was conducted. Northern General is a major medical care center for its region. It provides services to walk-in patients and accepts referrals from physicians in the surrounding communities and beyond. Some 70 percent of its patients are from the immediate urban area, 28 percent from the rest of the state in which it is located, and the remainder from the greater United States and even outside the country. They are drawn to Northern by the reputation of the hospital and its staff.

The hospital provides an impressive array of health care services. Its Emergency Room (ER) alone treats over 100,000 patients a year. Next door to the ER is a Primary Care Center (PCC) where regular patients come to see their assigned physicians for routine checkups and minor procedures. In the building rising over the ER and the PCC are housed many clinics for outpatient services—Eye Clinic, Radiation Clinic, Dental Clinic, and others. In the basement below, there is the Poison Control Center, a Rape Crisis Center, and a Cancer Hotline.

The hospital also has a special staff which deals with child and spouse abuse. And these are only outpatient services, provided to people who are not staying overnight in the hospital. The inpatient floors rising beyond the clinics, in several buildings, house nearly 1,000 patients and the nurses who support their basic medical care in surgical, pediatric, internal medicine, obstetrics and gynecology, psychiatric, and other specialties. The hospital, of course, owns CAT scanners, MRI devices, a linear accelerator, and what are now the entire array of technologies. Pediatricians here treat relatively rare diseases such as Reye's syndrome and Cooley's anemia, and the hospital boasts one of the nation's oldest and most renowned Newborn Intensive Care Units.

With such magnificent facilities, it is no wonder that Northern General is a major training center for physicians, nurses, technicians, and other health care workers. It is one of the 900 or so "teaching hospitals" in the nation directly affiliated with a major medical school.[2] There is a steep hierarchy of physicians, typical of such hospitals. The medical staff includes, first, senior physicians who hold positions as professors in the university's medical school as well as physicians from the community. These doctors are the "attending" physicians of the hospital and hold the top rank in the medical hierarchy. Just below the attendings are "Fellows," doctors at an advanced stage of training in specialized fields such as renal disease or endocrinology. Below these come the "house staff." They are employed by the hospital, not by the patients, as attendings are, and they work long hours (thirty-six-hour shifts perhaps twice a week, twelve hours other days). House staff are physicians, M.D.s, who are still in training; they are also called "residents." In their first year of training residents are usually called "interns." Most of the day-to-day medical decision making in the hospital is in the hands of the house staff; they are the physicians who are in the hospital handling the emergencies that come up at any time of the day or night.

The nursing administration is larger but a bit simpler. All nurses are employed by the hospital, and the nursing hierarchy

2. David Mechanic, *Medical Sociology*, 2d ed. (New York: Free Press, 1978), p. 374.

performs a large part of the hospital's administrative work. At the top of the Northern General nursing staff is a vice president for nursing of the hospital; below her are a half-dozen directors of nursing for different medical services of the hospital, for example, pediatrics, internal medicine, surgical nursing, etc. The next level is of supervisors who oversee a number of discrete floors or units. Each "floor" consists of a number (probably twenty to thirty) of patient beds and is headed by a head nurse. The head nurse, like a foreman of a work crew, directs the work of the bedside, or "staff," nurses. There are perhaps twenty to forty staff nurses under each head nurse, divided into three shifts (or two twelve-hour shifts in some ICUs). There are some twenty-five floors and a half-dozen units making up the hospital. The head nurse has the immediate daily responsibility for the floor or unit (the generic term for Intensive Care Units). Finally, at the bottom there are nursing students from the university's nursing school, who study for four years to receive a Bachelor of Science degree in nursing. Students typically will work in the hospital for one or two days a week, devoting the rest of their time to classroom studies. While working in the hospital, they usually care for a smaller number of patients than the full-time staff nurse, but the student nurse may well have many of the same responsibilities and tasks that a full-time R.N. does.

Physically, hospital floors look much like those on television soap operas: long hallways with rooms on either side, with the halls intersecting at a nurses' station, a configuration of boothlike desks behind which are clerks and nurses filling out the forms, answering the telephones, checking computer monitors, and taking care of the endless administrative tasks which consume as much of the nurse's time as does patient care. There is also a vast array of supplies and materials. On the desks in the nurse's station are polyurethane stackable boxes holding dozens and dozens (fifty or more) of multicopy forms for ordering all sorts of tests and procedures, billing forms, permission forms, order forms. On supply shelves, stacked to the ceiling, or jamming closets, or filling the walls of a pantry-like room in the hall, are adhesive tape, packaged needles, boxes of syringes, from 1 cubic centimeter (tiny), to 30, 40, 50 cc (a huge thing, the size of a baby's arm, used to deliver food in tube feedings), stacks of sterile isolation gowns in plastic wrappers, rubber bands, blood pressure cuffs, plastic jugs of microbial soap, bottles of saline solution, swabs, scales (for weighing patients' stools), large red plastic disposal jugs for used needles, plastic garbage bags, packaged kits of needles, sterile paper, syringes, and medications for doing lumbar puncture procedures, Foley urinary catheter insertion kits, intravenous kits, arterial catheter lines, and on, and on. The range and volume of visible, usable, disposable equipment is astonishing.

In the Intensive Care Units the equipment is multiplied with red "crash carts" carrying defibrillating machines and the wide range of drugs used for cardiac resuscitation; bottles of drugs like atropine, sodium bicarbonate, and epinephrine wedged into boxes on the fronts of patients' doors, ready to be used in an instant to juice up a failing heart; ring binders, several for each patient, with records of everything that is done to or for him or her. The equipment, the forms, the variety of supplies in themselves reflect the complexity of the organizations in which they are used, which provide and use them. Hospitals are complex, hierarchial organizations, and in that sense are like many other organizations in our society.

HOW THE HOSPITAL IS DIFFERENT

Much here is the same as in other organizations: the daily round of paper processing, answering the phone, making staffing decisions, collecting bills, ordering supplies, stocking equipment rooms; there are fights between departments, arguments with the boss, workers going home tired or satisfied. And medical sociology has made much of these similarities, using its research to create broader theories of, for instance, deviance or of the structure of professions.

But in one crucial respect the hospital remains dramatically different from other organizations: *in hospitals, as a normal part of the routine, people suffer and die.* This is unusual. "[A] good working definition of a hospital is that place where death occurs and no one notices; or, more sharply, the place where others agree to notice death as a social fact only so far as it fits their particular purposes."[3] Only combat military forces share this feature. To be complete, theories of hospital life need to acknowledge this crucial difference, since adapting themselves to pain and death is for hospital workers the most distinctive feature of their work. It is that which most separates them from the rest of us. In building theories of organizational life, sociologists must try to see how hospitals resemble other organizations—indeed, eventually that is what I am trying to do in this book—but we should not make a premature leap to the commonalities before appreciating the unique features of hospitals that make a nurse's task so different from that of a teacher or a businessman or a bureaucrat.[4]

A quick survey of typical patients in one Surgical Intensive Care Unit on one Saturday evening should make the point. The words in brackets are additions to my original field notes:

> *Room 1.* 64-year-old white woman with an aortic valve replacement; five separate IMEDs [intravenous drip-control devices] feeding in nitroglycerine, vasopressors, Versed [a pain killer which also blocks memory]. Chest tube [to drain off fluids]. On ventilator [breathing machine], Foley [catheter in the bladder], a pulse oximeter on her finger, a[rterial monitoring] line. Diabetic. In one 30-second period during the night, her blood pressure dropped from 160/72 to 95/50, then to 53/36, before the nurse was able to control the drop. N[urse]s consider her "basically healthy."
>
> *Room 2.* Man with pulmonary atresia, pulmonary valvotomy [heart surgery].
>
> *Room 3.* Woman with CABG [coronary artery bypass graft; a "bypass operation"]. Bleeding out [i.e., hemorrhaging] badly at one point during the night, they sent her back to the OR [Operating Room]. On heavy vasopressors [to keep blood pressure up].
>
> *Room 4.* Older woman with tumor from her neck up to her temple. In OR from 7 A.M. until 2 A.M. the next morning having it removed. Infarct [dead tissue] in the brain.

3. Bosk, *Forgive and Remember*, p. 90.

4. On the routinization of dying, see David Sudnow, *Passing On: The Social Organization of Dying* (Englewood Cliffs, NJ: Prentice-Hall, 1967).

> *Room 5.* 23-year-old woman, MVA [motor vehicle accident].
> ICP [intracranial pressure—a measure of brain swelling] mea-
> sured—terrible. Maybe organ donor. [Patient died next day.]
> *Room 6.* Don't know.
> *Room 7.* Abdominal sepsis, possibly from surgery. DNR [Do
> Not Resuscitate] today.
> *Room 8.* Big belly guy [an old man with a horribly distended
> abdomen, uncontrollable. Staff says it's from poor sterile tech-
> nique in surgery by Doctor M., who is notoriously sloppy. This
> patient died within the week.] [Field Notes]

This is a typical patient load for an Intensive Care Unit.
Eight beds, three patients dead in a matter of days. "Patients
and their visitors often find the ICU to be a disturbing, even
terrifying place. Constant artificial light, ceaseless activity, frequent emergencies, and the ever-present threat of death create
an atmosphere that can unnerve even the most phlegmatic
of patients. Some are so sick that they are unaware of their
surroundings or simply forget the experience, but for others
the ICU is a nightmare remembered all too well."[5] On
floors—the larger, less critical care wards of the hospital—
fatalities are less common, and patients are not so sick; even
so, one-third of the patients may have AIDS, another one-third
have cancer, and the rest suffer a variety of serious if not
immediately lethal diseases. The ICUs just get patients whose
deaths are imminent.

It is interesting that this density of disease presents one of
the positive attractions of nursing. People don't become nurses
to avoid seeing suffering or to have a quiet day. Every day
nurses respond to and share the most intense emotions with
total strangers. "People you don't know are going through the
most horrible things, and you are supposed to help them.
That's intense," says one nurse. And another enthuses about
coming home as the sun is coming up; the rest of the world
thinks things are just starting, and here you're coming off a
big emergency that lasted half the night: "[T]here's a real

---

5. Arnold S. Relman, "Intensive Care Units: Who Needs Them?" *New England
Journal of Medicine* 302 (April 1980), p. 965.

adrenaline kick in all this stuff. If you deny that, you're denying a big part of [nursing]."

The abnormality of the hospital scene liberates the staff from some niceties of everyday life and allows them a certain freedom. This will be treated in much fuller detail later in this book, but for now, two small, even silly, examples may illustrate the point. (1) Many nurses wear scrub suits—the pajama-like pants and tops worn in operating rooms and on some units. Written on the suits are phone numbers, vital statistics, or even doodles drawn during surgery. It's more convenient than finding a piece of paper. One observer, Judith André, has commented, "It's like a childhood fantasy" to scribble things on your clothes. (2) During a "code," as a patient was being resuscitated, one nurse who was having her period began to leak menstrual fluid. She ran into the patient's bathroom to change her sanitary pad. When she came out, another nurse, seeing the stain on her pants, yelled, "Well, J. got her period!"—a comment unthinkable in the everyday world. But this isn't the everyday world. As Everett Hughes wrote, "All occupations—most of all those considered professions and perhaps those of the underworld—include as part of their very being a licence to deviate in some measure from common modes of behavior."[6] In this sense, the hospital is like a war zone, in which common niceties and rules of decorum are discarded in the pursuit of some more immediate, desperate objective. There is an excitement, and a pressure, that frees hospital workers in the "combat zone" from an array of normal constraints on what they say and do.

And yet, for them their work has become normal, routine. On a medical floor, with perhaps two-thirds of the patients suffering eventually fatal diseases, I say to a nurse, "What's happening?" and she replies, walking on down the hall, "Same ol' same ol'." Nothing new, nothing exciting. Or in an Intensive Care Unit in the same hospital, "What's going on?" The resident replies, with a little shrug of the shoulders, "People are living, people are dying." Again, no surprises, nothing new. The routine goes on.

As other writers have noted, the professional treats rou-

6. Hughes, *Men and Their Work*, p. 79.

tinely what for the patient is obviously not routine. For the
health worker, medical procedures happen to patients every
day, and the hospital setting is quite comfortable: "The staff
nurse . . . belongs to a world of relative health, youth, and
bustling activity. She may not yet have experienced hospitalization herself for more than the removal of tonsils or the repair
of a minor injury. Although she works in an environment of
continuous sickness, she has been so conditioned to its external
aspects that she often expresses surprise when someone suggests that the environment must be anxiety evoking."[7] Everett
Hughes's formulation of this divergence of experience is classic: "In many occupations, the workers or practitioners . . .
deal routinely with what are emergencies to the people who
receive their services. This is a source of chronic tension between the two." Or, more precisely, "[O]ne man's routine of
work is made up of the emergencies of other people."[8]

To the patient, though, the hospital world is special, frightening, a jarring break from the everyday world. For the nurse,
it's just the "same ol' same ol'." How extreme the gap is was
observed in an ICU one evening:

> Three residents were attempting an LP [lumbar puncture—a
> "spinal tap" in which a long needle is inserted into the spinal
> column to draw out spinal fluid]. This is a very painful proce-
> dure and is difficult to perform. The television over the foot of
> the patient's bed was turned on, and "LA Law" was playing.
> While the resident was inserting the needle, she kept glancing
> up at the television, trying to simultaneously watch the show
> and do the LP. The patient, curled into the fetal position to
> separate the vertebrae, was unaware of this. The other two resi-
> dents as well were glancing back and forth from procedure to
> television. The resident tried for several minutes and was un-
> able to get the needle in properly, sometimes drawing out blood
> instead of fluid. Eventually, she called the head resident, who
> came in and successfully finished the LP. [Field Notes]

7. Esther Lucile Brown, "Nursing and Patient Care," in Fred Davis, *The Nursing Profession: Five Sociological Essays* (New York: John Wiley & Sons, 1966),
p. 202.

8. Hughes, *Men and Their Work*, pp. 54, 88.

This illustrates how casual staff can become, to the point of malfeasance.

How do staff, nurses in particular, routinize the abnormal? Or more fundamentally, what do we even mean by routinization?

WHAT ROUTINIZATION ENTAILS: THE OPERATING ROOM

The most egregious violation of commonsense morality—the profound physical violation of another person's body—is made completely routine in the hospital operating room. To help the reader understand routinization, we will consider this example in some detail.

In large teaching hospitals like Northern General or Southwest Regional, there are some twelve to twenty operating rooms in the "OR suite," with the rooms organized in a long hallway around a central equipment and supply area. The entire suite is "sterile," that is, everyone coming in and out wears scrub suits and face masks, shoe covers, and hair bonnets. Each operating room is furnished with a narrow padded table on which the patient lies during surgery, as well as with huge movable overhead lights and rolling tables for equipment of all sorts. Certain rooms are typically reserved for cardiac, neurological, orthopedic, and other special types of surgery, and the peculiar equipment for each of these is always available in those rooms. There are also one or two "crash rooms," for emergency surgery of the sort associated with the automobile wrecks or shootings frequently seen in large urban medical centers. Each room may be scheduled for one to six operations in a day; several dozen surgeries are scheduled for the hospital each weekday morning, usually starting at 6:00 and running until 2:00 or so in the afternoon.

Nurses manage these rooms between operations, supervising the flow of patients and the resupply of equipment (sponges, surgical tools, clean linens, etc.), answering the telephone or intercom and letting the physicians know when it is time to begin. There are typically at least two such nurses, the "scrub nurse" who assists the surgeon, handing tools and dealing directly with the sterile field, and the "circulating nurse" who can move in and out of the OR, touch nonsterile areas (such as the telephone), and keep the supplies flowing as needed to the surgical team. The circulating nurse is a kind of stage manager and fills in as needed, solving problems arising outside the surgery itself.

During surgery, the circulating nurse has several duties. First, she must document everything that happens: the time when surgery begins, what specific procedures are being conducted, what personnel are participating, when the procedure is done and "closing" begins, and when the patient is wheeled out of the room. Working together with the scrub nurse, she repeatedly counts and recounts the number of "sponges" (absorbent pads) used in the operation (there may be dozens). She must account for all of them both before and after the operation, to ensure that none are mistakenly left in the patient's body. She does the same for the surgical needles used, making certain that all are accounted for and disposed of properly, a serious concern since the advent of AIDS. The best circulating nurses, it would seem, are precise to the point of obsessiveness. The scrub nurse shares in these duties, counting sponges and accounting for all equipment, as well as passing to the surgeon, quickly and reliably, the specific tools needed at different stages of the operation. The scrub nurse also "preps" the patient: she drapes the patient with sterile cloths, leaving bare then shaving the area to be cut open, disinfecting the body surface with an iodine solution, and covering the skin with a clear plastic film called "Opsite" which protects the uncut area. A screen of cloth is usually set up between the patient's head and the rest of the body, so conscious patients will not see what's going on. This also means that the operating area is detached from the patient as a person, an important feature of the scene. The nurses carry out routine tasks dozens of times in a single day—for instance, the one-by-one counting of sponges, carried with tongs from a table to a waste bucket, perhaps two dozen of them counted aloud. The failure to perform these tasks conscientiously could be disastrous.

Once both room and patient are "prepped," the medical team can begin. The patient's body, fundamentally, is transformed into an object. An anesthesiologist (a physician), or a nurse anesthetist, will administer either a spinal anesthetic, which numbs the body below the injection point on the spinal cord, or a general anesthetic, which puts the patient to sleep. From then on, the operative area, screened from the patient's head and deadened of all feeling, effectively becomes to the surgeons a piece of nonhuman meat. The target area is isolated and immobilized; the patient is either asleep or, with a spinal, may be chatting away up at the head of the table with the anesthesiologist. In one case, a man's leg was being removed at one end of the table while at the other he was telling the anesthesiologist about his recent vacation trip. Looking at the operating area, the skin being cut or bone being sawed, you think, "No one I know has ever looked like this." Anesthetized flesh doesn't respond as the flesh of a living human being would. In amputations, the flesh being removed is usually dead and looks it—dark, hard, lifeless. But living flesh, too, on the table, looks more like what it "objectively" is, that is, meat. Human fat looks like the chicken fat you see on the stove; human skin peels back the way a chicken's does when peeled. An old man's tanned skin, when cut, looks like leather—which, precisely speaking, it is: old, tanned, animal skin. Surgeons working inside the body cavity remind one of cooks stuffing the Thanksgiving turkey, pulling open a section here, pushing a hand deep inside, feeling around for something there, stretching back tendons, trimming the fat, snipping pieces here and there with a small pair of scissors. The fine details of surgery are remarkably complex and refined, but its basic principles are brutally simple:

> To amputate this diabetic lady's toes, Dr. R., a small woman, used a thing like a big pair of bolt cutters to actually cut the bones, one toe at a time—with the big toe she had some difficulty, and she was almost lifted off the floor squeezing the big handles together before the "crunch" and the blades snapped through the toe. Then the last flesh was snipped away and five toes, all together, like a section of beef or chicken, came off in a single piece, and the scrub nurse laid it into a specimen tray. [Field Notes]

This primitive business is executed with simple tools: a razor-edge knife to cut open the skin (the scalpel); scissors to trim away flesh inside the body; smooth hooks to pull back the skin while the operation is underway (retractors); needle-nose pliers to shut off blood vessels (hemostats); and a small electric probe, essentially a soldering iron, used to cauterize the open ends of small blood vessels (the "Bovie"). Tools come in many sizes and specialized shapes, but this is the basic array. Orthopedic surgery adds its various saws, drills, and bits; the equipment table looks like a bench in an immaculate hobbyist's workshop, which in a sense it is.

To the senior staff, these tools and their uses become commonplace. During one routine orthopedic operation (routine for the staff, not for the patient), a group of young residents were working on a teenage patient's shoulder. The supervising attending physician, nominally in charge, popped in occasionally during the three-hour operation to see how things were going. On one visit he stopped for fifteen minutes to flip through the "swimsuit issue" of *Waterski* magazine, which one of the residents had brought. His pointed air of "no big deal" was more than casual; it seemed almost an assertion of his own power and sophistication, contrasted with the barely concealed anxiety of the residents he was monitoring. When he left, the residents visibly relaxed and resumed openly discussing how to perform the operation. One actually shuttled back and forth to a table against the wall to look at the diagrams in his textbook to see how the surgery should be done. Then the attending anesthesiologist came in to check on his resident and to sign a form ("So I'll get my cut," he said smiling) and walked out again. Music by popular musicians Phil Collins and Los Lobos was on a portable tape cassette player as the residents worked. The residents were learning to do highly skilled surgery and how to regard it as part of everyday life.

Routinization in the OR or elsewhere in the hospital seems to mean several things: that actions are repeated, that they violate normal taboos, and that routine is embedded in behavior. Consider each in turn, drawing on further examples from other settings in the hospital:

1. *Repeatability.* Each operation is not the first of its kind; most in fact are done several times each day and hundreds of times each year, even by a single team of surgeons, nurses, and technical aides. What the team sees, they have seen many times. Gallbladder removals, hernia repairs and shoulder operations

on athletes—these are all very common procedures in the major medical center.[9]

And those repeated procedures take place against the even less dramatic background of the repeated daily events of the nurse's work: starting intravenous lines, taking blood pressures four times a day on every patient on the floor, drawing blood samples, charting vital signs, writing nurses' progress notes, passing food trays, helping patients on and off the bedpan. Both trivial and consequential activities are repeated over and over until each one becomes much like the next; indeed, as Hughes says, the professional's "very competence comes from having dealt with a thousand cases of what the client likes to consider his unique experience."[10] Says one nurse, "You get to the point where you don't really care for the patients anymore, and one GI [gastrointestinal] bleeder gets to be the same as the next GI bleeder."

In a Medical Intensive Care Unit, death itself becomes an often-repeated event:

> Another MICU patient just coded and died; that's five in the past six days. Incredible. The docs are here one month— N[urse]s are here for good . . .
> I just came in unit; first N[urse] says, "You just missed it." They said that to me a few days ago. It's not that I "just miss," I think, but rather that so much [is] going on. You'll always "just miss" something. [Field Notes]

Death becomes a routinized part of daily life, incorporated into the flow. "Mr. Smith died last night," says one nurse to another. "Oh, that's too bad. He was such a nice man"; a casual exchange. One day is like another, if not for Mr. Smith, then at least for the rest of us. For the nurses Mr. Smith will be replaced by another man, a Mr. Jones, with similar ailments

---

9. Some physicians have astonishing numbers of routinized operations to their credit. For example, Dr. Denton Cooley of Houston has performed over 75,000 open heart surgeries with his team. Over two-thirds were personally performed by Dr. Cooley. *Guinness Book of World Records* New York: Bantam Books, 1988).

10. Hughes, *Men and Their Work,* p. 54.

and a similar end. Like the fictional prep school teacher Mr. Chips, for whom the students "never get older," nurses see the same patients over and over, even if the names change.

> On Infant Unit: "He [baby] looks better."
> "Yeah, 'he looks better': Baby Watson, Baby Jackson . . ." (two infants who were here for a long time, up and down, eventually Watson died—Jackson is still here, 9 months, hopeless).
> "Why can't they just come in sick and bleeding, look bad, and go?" (die immediately without the emotional ups and downs).
> Above said by two nurses on ISCU [Infant Special Care Unit] one night while working. [Field Notes]

The repeatability of the events—the sense that the same things happen over and over—is part of what is meant by routinization.

2. *Profanation.* Normally, we experience our bodies and the bodies of others as sacred, as areas to be approached with reverence or even with awe. To the healthy person outside the hospital, the body is special, a thing distinct from other things in the world, and must be treated as different. Physical contact with other bodies is emotionally provocative, in ways good and bad. A touch, a hug, a kiss arouse some sensitivity; a slap, however light, provokes humiliation or perhaps rage. But for patients in the hospital, their bodies are dramatically profaned. The body is often exposed to strangers, older and younger, male and female, even in groups. Many times a day the patient's body is punctured by injection needles. It is the object of teachers' lectures to their students. It is touched frequently, often without special preliminaries. It is probed with fingers and hands and tools in ways that are sometimes brutal, with little respect for the body as a sacred object. Even when professionals are respectful (and many of them always are), the effect on patients is one of secularization of their own flesh. Anne Sexton says in her poem "The Operation,"

> Clean of the body's hair,
> I lie smooth from breast to leg.
> All that was special, all that was rare

is common here. Fact: death too is in the egg.
Fact: the body is dumb, the body is meat.[11]

   The profanation of the sexual parts in particular is profound in medical settings, despite the elaborate preliminaries
of draping the patient, and the like: "All that was special . . .
is common here."[12] Earlier in Sexton's poem, in an examination, the patient found herself having to "allow the glove its
oily rape." Gynecological examinations have been the subject
of excellent studies of the construction of realities.[13] Similar
work could be done on the three-second prostate exams (often
preceded by a none-too-comforting "This is going to hurt");
proctoscopy and sigmoidoscopy (which entail insertion of a
hollow tube into the rectum and colon); and cystoscopy (examination of the bladder through a tube into the urethra). Perhaps
more than other invasive "lookings," such as bronchoscopy,
these invasions of the private parts can be humiliating to the
patient. One nurse reports that the most difficult thing she
witnessed in nursing school was an episiotomy made before
childbirth, as she and her classmates audibly gasped when they
heard the scissors click down; identification with the patient
was unavoidable. For a male observer a different scene has a
similar effect.

> Patient under a general [anesthetic], in for leg amputation.
> Nurse putting in a Foley (urinary) catheter, first scoured the
> end of the penis, foreskin pulled back, with a series of three
> pads soaked in Betadine. Rapid circular motion . . . Then lifting
> the penis and, with a pair of disposable pliers holding the cathe-
> ter, threading it into the urethra, pushing it all the way in up

11. Anne Sexton, *All My Pretty Ones* (Cambridge, MA: Riverside Press, 1961),
p. 13.
12. "I see a lot of crotches," says one nurse. "Old ladies: 'I have to wash your
privates, dear.' Then some of them lock their legs together, others just spread
'em wide. And young guys, twenty years old, you start cleaning and they get
hard. I think that's tough for them." [Field Notes]
13. Joan Emerson, "Behavior in Private Places: Sustaining Definitions of Reality in Gynecological Examinations," in Hans Peter Dreitzel, *Recent Sociology No.
2: Patterns of Communicative Behavior* (New York: Macmillan Company, 1970),
pp. 73–101.

to the bladder, fast. There seemed to be resistance, but she just pushed on. More than matter-of-fact, completely mechanical. No gentleness to it. I was glad the patient was unconscious. [Field Notes]

While the patient lies suffering in a bed, the staff carries on, and the rest of the world goes about its business with no evident reverence. And the ever-present television provides a steady background, perhaps just like home, importing the banality of everyday life into the heart of the least banal settings:

> *Bizarre scene, but typical:* 5:30 A.M. in the ICU. In bed in room 7 is Mr. L., with a bka [below the knee amputation] of the leg . . . TV over his bed is on, an aerobics show. Three women in red leotards with electric blue tights and ankle weights, all smiles, jumping with arms up, spinning, clapping hands, stamping feet to the music. It's upbeat, happy, "wake up, everybody!" Next room is AIDS patient with bp [blood pressure] 91/48, 4 IV poles, 8 bags of fluids going in, on a ventilator. As the nurses work, they often glance up, watching the TV. [Field Notes]

Even in the presence of visitors, nurses can be remarkably oblivious to the way they ignore daily taboos. A nurse walking through the unit, where patients' friends and family are sitting in most of the rooms, calls out to a colleague, "Is room 1 a No Code?"—in other words, Will we let her die? Here, it seems, nothing is sacred.

3. *Existentiality.* Routinization of the abnormal involves not so much a mental leap as an existential action; creating a routine is not some trick of the conscious mind but rather a whole way of acting that involves physical as well as mental components. It comprises embodied habits. Routinization is not "all in the head"; it is something one does. It is carried out in the way a nurse walks and talks while in the presence of abnormal events. It entails that "matter of factness" with which she inserts a bladder catheter or cleans up feces; it is evidenced in the full range of emotions she shows, laughing with a dying man, chatting and even laughing with colleagues during a code (a resuscitation effort), glancing casually through a nursing journal filled with full-color advertisements for ileostomy ap-

pliances and crèmes for cancer lesions. After a middle-aged woman died late one night in room 5 of a medical ICU, her family, loudly crying and hugging each other, came into the room to see their dead mother. Outside the room, three nurses who had tried for thirty minutes to resuscitate the patient sat around a table eating corn chips and gossiping, as if nothing had happened. One of those nurses said to me, "We're pretty dehumanized, huh?" but it wasn't true: if she were dehumanized, no such comment would even be made. She knew what was happening, and eating corn chips, even then, is in fact quite human. In a unit where three patients die each week, to get upset with every death would be humanly unacceptable.

So in the Operating Room and elsewhere events are repeated over and over, in an attitude of secularized treatment of the body, and this repeated attitude is built into and expressed in the very ordinary doings of the staff. Sometimes routinization goes beyond mere commonplace into an attitude of detachment, unconcern, or sheer boredom—one of the more common emotions of the nurse's life, to the surprise of laypersons. Indeed, one of the most frequent questions nurses asked me during my research was, "Aren't you bored?" It was asked at least two or three times a week, in different settings— perhaps most strangely in the very busy ICUs:

> "Don't you get bored?" JD, a n[urse] in the ICU, asked me tonight while sitting outside rooms 1-4: man w/CA [cancer]; man w/AIDS, who's a No Code; Mr. Watkins, who's been here four months, ventilator dependent, no hope; woman w/encephalitis, shaking [in convulsions] all the time—none of them awake and aware. No, I said. She said, "Do you get enough ethics stuff?" [Field Notes]
>
> N[urse] in ICU today asks, "Aren't you bored?" I laughed, said, "Take two steps back and look around. I'm not a nurse." She paused, looked around, and started laughing. Understood. [Field Notes]

Nurses themselves, especially those in intensive care and emergency settings, need what one calls their "crisis fix" each day. They want to work with the desperately ill or injured; they thrive on the excitement of the crash room and the code.

The first time one deals with the victim of a motorcycle accident, everything is new and demanding, but after one or two each weekend, the routine sets in. Without continuing new challenges, even surgery, dramatic or even catastrophic to the patient, can become a boring routine. As one OR scrub nurse said between surgeries one day,

> I'm sick of boobs [mastectomies], I'm sick of colies [cholecystectomies—gall bladder removals], I'm sick of hernias. I want some fun cases. [Field Notes]

HOW ROUTINIZATION IS ACCOMPLISHED: CREATING CONDITIONS FOR ORDINARY LIFE

Thus, for the nurse, hospital life is ordinary—not extraordinary, or mystical, or even an object of thoughtful scrutiny. We saw in the last section how the nurse's ordinary daily life consists largely of repeated, secular activities. Things happen, time and time again, in essentially the same way; these happenings are for the most part devoid of any special, sacred character; and they are carried out in the working world, through concrete actions, not merely (or not even) thought about in any conscious way. "The ambience of nursing units is not tragic, but mundane and businesslike. The work of nurses and aides is largely repetitive and is carried on largely in a habitual manner . . . For the most part, nursing personnel seem to be hardly perturbed at the graphic condition of their patients . . . When they enter the presence of a sorely afflicted patient, their countenances are not likely to betray more than a flicker of emotion."[14] This is what we mean by saying the nurse has routinized the world of the hospital. Her life here has taken on a quality of mundane sameness, often to the point of sheer boredom.

> The first time I had to interview a patient in my first year of nursing school, he said he had a scar [on his chest]. I asked to see it, he just pulled up his gown [around his neck; she gestures to show how he was bare]. I was . . . [rolls her eyes, embar-

14. Ronald Philip Preston, *The Dilemmas of Care: Social and Nursing Adaptions to the Deformed, the Disabled and the Aged* (New York: Elsevier, 1979), p. 93.

rassment] "Oh, my God." And now . . . [waves her hand, flutters eyes to indicate her totally blasé attitude]. [Field Notes]

No lay person would experience such exposure so casually. And nudity is simple; witnessing open heart surgery, or an endotracheal intubation, or CPR, is far more threatening to one's everyday reality. But nurses see these events every day, without becoming upset. The nurse's view—or more accurately, the nurse's very way of *living* here and dealing with such trauma—is different from ours.

How does this casual attitude develop? How does the abnormal become routine? The conventional answer is that "you just get used to it." This implies that over time, with enough exposure, one adapts, willy-nilly, to whatever is happening in the environment. This may be true, but it is insufficient. "Getting used to it" suggests that routinization is purely a matter of the passage of time, with repetition as the implied causative agent. Yes, routinization happens "over time," but time alone is insufficient to cause routinization. Some nurses never become accustomed, as we will see, to deformed newborns, or psychotic teenagers, or incontinent geriatric patients. Then, too, some people "get used to it" virtually immediately. Before my own first witnessing of surgery, I conscientiously followed all the head nurse's instructions to avoid physical or emotional upset: I rose early, ate a full breakfast, and was wide awake before going to the OR suite. After donning the scrub suit, bonnet, and shoe covers, I went into the OR and asked the circulating nurse what the first case would be, hoping for something "easy," maybe a wrist or ankle operation. She looked at the chart and said, without missing a beat, "leg amputation." I nearly panicked, but I stayed. To my own amazement, I was not in the least upset by the amputation or any of the surgeries I witnessed, including the repair of a ruptured ectopic pregnancy that drove at least two experienced nurses from the OR in dismay. For some reason, there seemed to be no period of "getting used to it" at all. So repeated exposure as a means of routinization is insufficient; more is at work.

At least four phenomenological tasks go into the routinization of the hospital world: learning one's geographical surroundings, so that the routine is physically manageable; learning the language so one can meet and work with other people; learning the technique of the work being done (if you don't know how to start an IV, it's hard to be casual about it); and learning the "types" of patients and the standard procedures for recognizing and dealing with them. Each of these four steps seems to be involved when nurses talk about "getting used to it." There is also, harder to define, a fifth task, a perceptual "leap," which I will describe after presenting these components. Together these produce a sense of ordinariness, both cognitive and behavioral:

> The ordinariness of the world is socially produced . . .
> People are constantly engaging in cognitive practices to make the world ordinary, to treat whatever happens as if it were just another instance of something familiar and commonsensical. The fact that we have successfully made our experiences ordinary keeps us from seeing how we did it . . .[15]

While largely invisible to those living it, ordinariness, I think, can nevertheless be explicated. Consider the five tasks in turn:

1. *Learning the geography.* The first step in the routinization of a world is simply to learn one's way around the physical setting. It's difficult to be casual when rooms are unfamiliar, hallways look long and forbidding, and one can't find the bathroom. Supplies are often kept in unexpected places, telephones sometimes work in strange ways ("You have to dial 8 first"), even chairs may have traditional claims on them (until recently in American hospitals, nurses stood while physicians sat). Hospital beds come in various models, and working them isn't always easy.

This geography has social meanings and implications, too, which must be learned. One has to know that "this is Joanne's chair," or that the clerk always gets the phone, or that everyone cleans their own coffee cup. The physical setting, that is, must be known in its social ramifications. Again, perhaps my own experience is not unusual:

---

15. Randall Collins, *Theoretical Sociology* (New York: Harcourt Brace Jovanovich, 1988), p. 279.

My sensitivity is going; I'm getting used to the hospital. The strangeness of the people who work there—nurses, aides, orderlies, maids, doctors—is fading, as they fall neatly into these groups, and as I come to understand what these people and statuses mean in the hospital. It scares me less; I no longer feel discomfort at the rooms full of tubes and bottles and complicated beds of cranks and pulleys. I am no longer embarrassed by disease. Cartons of medicine, not colorful but white cartons, with red and black lettering in words that end in -in and -ex, boxes of disposable hypodermic needles. This is the nurse's world . . . The nurses live here 8 hours a day and use this space and these things; these belong to them; the surgeon has the operating room, but these wards belong to the nurses, and it is from here that they run the hospital. It is their home territory, where they are as comfortable as anywhere. They often can't understand, although they are aware of, the outsider's fear of this place . . . for them it is all normal . . . Entering the nurse's world is more than a physical act . . . Rooms come to have meanings, significance; some rooms you come to like, some to fear and despise. No floor map can show you these things. [Field Notes]

2. *Learning the language.* To move easily in the world of the hospital, the nurse must learn its peculiar language, the technical jargon, and the informal slang. The jargon is technically complex, even daunting. DNR: an order to Do Not Resuscitate a terminal patient when his or her breathing or heartbeat stops. CABG: pronounced "Cabbage," a coronary artery bypass graft, what the layperson calls bypass surgery. Or consider this description of the possible causes of one common symptom.

[It is found] accompanying diaphragmatic pleurisy, pneumonia, uremia, or alcoholism . . . abdominal causes include disorders of the stomach, and esophagus, bowel diseases, pancreatitis, pregnancy, bladder irritation, hepatic metastases, or hepatitis. Thoracic and mediastinal lesions or surgery may be responsible. Posterior fossa tumors or infarcts may stimulate centers in the medulla oblongata . . .[16]

16. *The Merck Manual of Diagnosis and Therapy,* 15th ed. (Rahway, NJ: Merck Sharp & Dohme Research Laboratories, 1987), pp. 1356–1357.

Pity the poor layperson who overhears such language to discuss his or her symptom—which in this case is hiccups.

Besides medical jargon, informal slang is highly developed, as the staff live in an experiential world far different than the layperson. Here, a dying patient is "going down the tubes," "circling the drain." The dead have "bought the farm," "straight-lined," or perhaps "Marshalled"—a reference to the name of the building that houses the morgue. An older patient who violently resists the nurses is "confused" and after drug sedation becomes much more "appropriate." Every emergency room has its "Gomers"—one of the most ubiquitous cases of hospital slang, derived from "Grand Old Man of the ER," or variants, and referring generically to old people with no treatable problems who are virtually permanent residents of the hospital.[17] On the acute psychiatric unit, there is the "quiet room": what once was called a padded cell, where a suicidal teenage girl huddles in a corner, crying, visible through the peephole in the door. The patient is regularly technicized in discussions of "input" and "output" (of food and waste). Learning the peculiar language is a vital part of becoming an insider. To understand what people are talking about, much less to become comfortable here, you need to learn the slang.[18] And even when no special jargon is used, the very matter-of-factness of the talk can be disarming: "Well, he had a stool; it was soft, but he said there was some diarrhea." Most of us simply don't talk in that way with fellow workers.

3. *Learning the techniques.* Routinization requires learning the techniques of one's work: the job itself must be familiar. One reason that I was immediately "used to" seeing surgery was that I was only observing it, not participating. Observing is a skill at which, as a sociologist, I have had much practice. There was no further technical learning necessary.

Nursing entails a great number of specific technical skills, and until one learns them the job can be overwhelming. "Being organized" is a prime job skill for nurses. The staff nurse dis-

---

17. See Samuel Shem, M.D., *The House of God* (New York: Dell Publishing Co., 1978), for many more examples.

18. "No profession can do its work without licence to talk in shocking terms about clients and their problems." Hughes, *Men and their Work,* p. 82.

penses hundreds of pills a day to dozens of patients, starts and maintains intravenous lines, gives bed baths, documents on paper virtually everything she does, monitors temperatures, blood pressures, and urine "outputs," delivers food trays, and responds more or less to all the miscellaneous patient and family requests that, from her point of view, often get in the way of her finishing her basic required work. Simply getting through an eight-hour shift without mistakenly giving Mrs. Jones the pills for Ms. Smith, or forgetting to check Mr. Martin's IV line, or not helping Miss Garcia eat her lunch is challenge enough. And these are the everyday, nonemergency tasks, the basics of the job. In the operating room, a circulating nurse is responsible for setting up tables with hundreds of small tools, stocking the correct combination of gauze sponges, suture kits, sterile gowns, and all the rest, knowing that surgeons are notoriously demanding; the scrub nurse sequentially passes the surgeon dozens of tools, when it matters most. Indeed, the mass of details that nurses organize can appear overwhelming. And each detail, so apparently innocuous, can have enormous implications—as when a single sponge, one out of dozens used, is left inside a patient after surgery, or when one wrong pill goes to a heavily medicated patient. Thus, outstanding nurses often are described as "really well organized." So one can admire the supervisor nurse who clearly commands her job:

> Rae Kelly sits at the phone in the unit, a steady flow of people standing in short lines, talking with her, while she never puts the phone down, only punching the buttons from one line to the other, and answering her beeper as well. Clerks, HNs[head nurses from other units] come by—almost no breaks for several hours this evening. Mostly concerning staffing [getting enough nurses in to work, sorting them to the units where most needed], she's supervising this section tonight. [Field Notes]

Not surprisingly, some of the techniques to be learned are in themselves morally problematic, modifying what one sees as decent or even acceptable ways of treating other human beings. At the mildest level, much medical therapy is notably "aggressive," using invasive procedures (such as surgery), massive doses of potent drugs, removal and replacement of a patient's blood, bone marrow, bodily organs, or even—in a different specialty—a human personality. It is not unusual for hospital patients to receive half a cupful of pills every morning, each of which produces a significant change in the body's functioning. Patients who normally receive one "needle stick" per year, say in a blood test or flu shot, will be stuck ten times every *day* in the hospital. And there are the enemas, limitation of liquids, repeated physical exams, and the like, all a routine part of the patient's experience. Such procedures are, no doubt, preferable to the patient's remaining ill, but many are "required" not so much by the disease as by the organizational inefficiency of the hospital (multiple blood tests are an obvious culprit here). And all are carried out, in person, by nurses, who thereby must modify most of their conventional notions of what people eat, how they sleep (not past 6:00 A.M.), and how bodies are to be treated.

Beyond that, nurses have developed an array of techniques for controlling recalcitrant patients. Much of Chapter Five will be devoted to the issue of "noncompliance" among patients. Here let us just note that the nurse must accommodate herself to the idea, if not the practice, of routinely using sedatives to control agitated patients ("But I won't do it," says one. "That's not what those drugs are for."); or of surgeons' using paralytic drugs when performing certain difficult procedures, or using memory blockers like Versed, realizing that patients won't remember what you had to do to them; or of restraining old people who would otherwise fall out of bed and break a hip. All of these practices are defensible, but they require a different view of acceptable practices than the outsider normally has. Nurses quickly learn that patients have to be managed, sometimes through physical or chemical restraints, for nurses to get their work done. After a while, nobody questions that all ventilator patients are restrained (tied down), that patients who pull out their IVs are similarly restrained, that most ICU patients are continually drugged, even when not in obvious pain, and that patients sleep and wake according to the hospital's schedule, not their own. Once a nurse accommodates herself to the practices, routinizes the techniques, learns to do them quickly and efficiently, the job isn't so overwhelming:

"You're quiet today, Dan," Lou said to me today, while writing at the nursing station desk.

"I don't want to interfere with your work."

"Nobody can interfere. We can listen to the phone, chart, and talk at the same time." [Field Notes]

4. *Learning the patients.* Patient types, too, become routine to the nurse. Despite an outsider's first impression of a multitude of different medical problems, most patients suffer one of a fairly small number of predictable ailments: cancer, heart disease, COPD (chronic obstructive pulmonary disease, such as emphysema or bronchitis), and now AIDS. These cover most of the severe cases. Treatments are relatively predictable as well, from the nursing staff's perspective: surgery, intravenous therapy, the usual medications. In heart disease, there are perhaps a half-dozen routinely used drugs; for cancer, there is surgery and the usual chemotherapy or radiation. So patients quickly become typed: the COPD lady in room 8, the AIDS guy in 2. And each of the floors or units has its typical crises:

> The E[mergency] R[oom] got a 35-year-old tonight—fell out of the back of a pickup truck. There were 2 of these during [a local festival]—one each weekend. And I saw another in the Neurosurg[ery] ICU last week. It's a [local] tradition.
>
> On Geri[atric floor] last night, they had a code [CPR]: old lady went to the bathroom, got sick and [cardiac] arrested. [Field Notes]
>
> In M[edical] ICU this morning, nurse yells down hall "Ellen, I'm gonna need your help, he just had a bowel movement."
>
> Laughter. "Oh my God, he got loose [from restraints]," says another.
>
> Laughter from several nurses heading to the room to take care of things. P[atient] g[astro]i[ntestinal] bleeder—drinks 12 beers a day, he says, down from 20 or more. [Later discover it's more like 30.] Shakes, tremors, DTs bad, huge swollen tight belly. One n[urse] changes the sheets, other checks to see if he's oriented—"What's your job? Where do you live?" [Field Notes]

These are typical patient problems in these units; the nurses are accustomed to them and know how to deal with them. They even have methods for dealing with obnoxious patients:

> Cardiac patient, middle-aged man. Screams "Goddamn!" loud, when nurse puts in needle for blood. He yells "Bedpan!" when he wants it. [This is a small unit; all patients around can hear this, if they aren't too drugged out.] One nurse says, "I think it's just his way of communicating. That's how I deal with it." Another says, with a smile, as she walks out of his room, "We have a personality conflict." [Patient died the next day.] [Field Notes]

An advantage of being used to seeing pain is that one can then work with suffering people. The "detached concern" that Robert Merton writes about allows a nurse to lose the embarrassment many of us feel in front of sick people and allows her to talk with sick or dying patients. A dying woman can tell a nurse her fears; she may hesitate to burden a friend with them. A nurse, one may believe, has seen it all, so seeing one more thing perhaps won't upset her. It's probably true. One nurse told me that a friend said to her, "My dad is on oxygen!" and she, the nurse, thought to herself, "What would these people think if they saw someone in the unit with IV lines, an NG [nasogastric] tube, chest tubes, a catheter stuck in the bladder, and another tube stuck up the rectum? Ye gods, everyone I *know* is on oxygen!" She has become familiar with patients.

Having learned the geography of the hospital, the language, the techniques of work, and the types of patient, a nurse is well prepared to convert what was a chaos of disasters into a routine, well-organized round of daily activities.

5. *Routinization of the world.* But learning the specifics of the job—the geography, the jargon, the techniques, the patients—does not automatically produce an acceptance of the hospital world as normal. Some nurses learn the techniques but still never accept the daily disasters; they leave the profession, or move to less acute care settings, working in a school, a physician's office, or perhaps a home health care agency. More is demanded than simply accruing new information about work, or people, or the setting. Routinization itself demands a qualitative transformation in one's thinking, an entirely new way of relating to events and people. It can happen

suddenly. Some nurses say that after six months or so on the job, having struggled through the heavy demands, often near to despair, one day they realize that the work no longer bothers them; they are "into" it.

> When I [first] walked into that unit, I had never seen any of these machines . . . there are 15,000 machines, they all have different alarms, they all have different ways to work them, different trouble-shooting things, and here you are expected to take care of this patient who's crumping every minute . . . it's just overwhelming. . .
>
> And then all of a sudden, one day, you say, Gee, I've survived this shift, and all of these things happened, and it was O.K. . . .
>
> [So what happened that you got used to it?]
>
> You know, I have absolutely no idea . . . You go in and you do it again and again, and your patient codes for the fifth time . . . I can't even tell you when it happens, it's different for different people . . .
>
> Then the scary thing happens. You start to *like* it. [Field Notes]

What this nurse describes is not just a gradual transition over time, not a simple accumulation of experiences that finally equal "getting used to it." The accumulation of experiences is part of it, to be sure. But these only make possible the major shift, a qualitative transformation of consciousness, a *routinization of the world*. It is as if one takes the proverbial journey of a thousand single steps and discovers that the final step is in fact a fifteen-foot jump over a deep mountain gorge. Without that final leap, the journey is incomplete, almost a waste. But even that analogy doesn't quite fit, since many nurses "jump the gorge" without ever realizing what they have done. Usually, it just happens ("How did you get used to it?" "I have absolutely no idea."). Still, it is the nurse who "does" this happening, who makes the leap, even if unconsciously.

Or to try another analogy: the nurse accepts the routine of the hospital much as a listener accepts the rhythm and flow of a formerly unfamiliar piece of music. You, the reader, may have sometime listened to the first few measures of a piece of music, or the first few notes, and for a moment you could not tell what was happening. It was a chaos of sound. Perhaps you couldn't discern the melody, or couldn't, for instance, in a jazz work, find the rhythm to which it was played; perhaps it was not even recognizable as an orderly composition at all. Some kinds of music (disco, for instance) have a pattern that is easy to find and follow; for others (jazz, especially) the patterns are relatively difficult and to the layperson perhaps impossible to understand. One must develop a feel for the music, probably over time, and then *give oneself over* to it. This is neither completely a function of the music itself nor of the listener; it is an interaction of the two. The listener must at some point take on the appropriate attitude to be able to hear what is happening in the piece. Similarly, a nurse must give herself to the rhythm of the hospital, must "get into" what is happening; she must accept its normality and take up its rhythms and melodies as her own. So the leap into a routine, where to the layperson there is chaos, cannot be impelled by all of the training that has come before. Routinization of this world (or any other) remains a free lived act of the individual.

Speaking more broadly of the coherent, normal "lifeworld" generally, philosopher Maurice Natanson has written, "The *Lebenswelt* [lifeworld] is a constituted reality dependent upon an immanent fiat of consciousness."[19] This means that routinization is (1) a "fiat," or what I have called a "leap" or qualitative transformation; and (2) while certain objective conditions, as I've described, set the stage for routinization, they cannot finally cause it to happen. An ICU may have three deaths a week in an eight-bed unit, with a calculable standard deviation from this mean on any given week. A sociologist can plot these rates and record what happens if the rate goes way over this norm. But normality is neither found in the objective state of things (what "usually" happens in the hospital) nor in the nurse's subjective feelings about them (e.g., she stops getting upset, doesn't care, feels "bored," etc.). Routinization is found instead in the way in which the nurse lives in the hospital—not just her thoughts and feelings but her very posture, in the broadest sense: how she walks down a hallway, how she

19. Maurice Natanson, *Phenomenology, Role, and Reason: Essays on the Coherence and Deformation of Social Reality* (Springfield, IL: Charles C. Thomas, 1974), p. 124.

converses with the patients, how she handles the tools of her trade. With sick people all around, what does the nurse do? She does her job, she reads a magazine, she smokes a cigarette. During rounds, she listens casually:

> Some of the patients discussed today in the morning staff meeting [on a surgical floor]:
> —high school boy who ran through a window, "spoiled kid, very demanding"
> —man with leg run over by fork lift
> —guy (23) with testicular cancer—spirits are good, though
> —woman who cut finger on lawn mower, now infected
> —man (28) with sudden blindness, probably caused by little strokes
> —woman who won't eat or drink, asks for IV; wants to stay in the hospital; considered very weird. [Field Notes]

During this meeting, nurses sip their coffee or whisper to their neighbors. Old issues of *Redbook* lie on the table next to the patients' medical charts. Strewn around the conference room are coffee cups (styrofoam or ceramic, often with names on them), a candy wrapper or two, an old softball schedule, and some plastic food utensils. The outsider's sense of dread, or dismay, at what is happening with patients has vanished; the mention of serious disease or death gets a nod, perhaps, but no more. Here in the hospital, to these nurses, terrible things have become ordinary.

TWO

Protecting the Routine
from Chaos

Every unit in the hospital, then, has its own normality, its own typical patients, number of deaths, and crises to be faced. But just as predictably, every unit has its emergencies that threaten the routine and challenge the staff's ability to maintain workaday attitudes and practices. Emergencies threaten the staff's ability to carry on as usual, to maintain their own distance from the patient's suffering, and to hold at bay their awe at the enormity of events. Occasionally breakdowns occur in unit discipline or the ability to do the required work.

Staff follow several strategies when trying to manage the threat of breakdowns: they will keep outsiders outside, follow routinization rituals, or use humor to distance themselves. Finally, even when all efforts fail, they will keep going, no matter what. Consider in turn each of these implicit maxims:

1. *Keep outsiders outside.* Every hospital has policies about visiting hours, designed not only to "let patients rest" but also to protect staff from outsiders' interference in their work. Visitors are limited to certain hours, perhaps two to a patient room for fifteen-minute visits; they may have to be announced before entering the unit or may be kept waiting in a room down the hall. No doubt many such policies are good for the patient. No doubt, too, they keep visitors out of the nurse's way, prevent too many obtrusive questions or requests for small services, and prevent curious laypersons from seeing the messier, less presentable sides of nursing care.

When visitors cannot be physically excluded, they can still be cognitively controlled, that is, prevented from knowing that something untoward is happening. Typically, the staff behave in such episodes as if everything were OK, even when it is not. This is similar to what Erving Goffman observed in conversations: when the shared flow of interaction is threatened by an accidental insult or a body failure such as a sneeze or flatulence, people simply try to ignore the break in reality and carry on as if nothing has happened. Such "reality maintenance" is often well-orchestrated, requiring cooperation on the part of several parties. For Goffman, normal people in normal interactions accept at face value each other's presentation of who they are:

> A state where everyone temporarily accepts everyone else's line is established. This kind of mutual acceptance seems to be a basic structural feature of interaction, especially the interaction of face-to-face talk. It is typically a "working" acceptance, not a "real" one.[1]

And when this routine breaks down, the immediate strategy is simple denial:

> When a person fails to prevent an incident, he can still attempt to maintain the fiction that no threat to face has occurred. The most blatant example of this is found where the person acts as if an event that contains a threatening expression has not occurred at all.[2]

In the hospital, the unexpected entrance of outsiders into a delicate situation can disrupt the staff's routine activities and create unmanageable chaos. To avoid this, the staff may pretend to outsiders that nothing special is happening; this pretense itself can be part of the routine. During a code (resuscitation) effort I witnessed, there were three such potential disruptions by outsiders: another patient calling for help, a new incoming patient being wheeled in, and the new patient's family members entering the unit. All three challenges were handled by the staff diverting the outsiders from the code with a show, as if nothing were happening:

> Code in CCU [Cardiac Care Unit] . . . woman patient, asystole [abnormal ventricle contractions]. Doc (res[ident]) pumping

1. Erving Goffman, "On Face-Work," in *Interaction Ritual: Essays on Face-to-Face Behavior* (New York: Pantheon Books, 1967), p. 11.
2. Ibid., pp. 17–18.

chest—*deep* pumps, I'm struck by how far down they push. Serious stuff. Matter of factness of process is striking. This was a surprise code, not expected. Patient was in Vtak [ventricular fibrillation], pulse started slowing, then asystole. N[urse]s pumping for a while, RT [Respiratory Therapist] ambu-bagging [pumping air into lungs]. Maybe 7–8 people in patient's room working. Calm, but busy. Occasionally a laugh.

Pt in next room (no more than 10 feet away) called for nurse—a doc went in, real loose and casual, strolled in, pt said something; doc said, "There's something going on next door that's taking people's time; we'll get to you"—real easy, like nothing at all happening. Then strolls back to code room. Very calm . . .

Two N[urse]s came into unit wheeling a new patient. One said, "Uh, oh, bad time," very quietly as she realized, going in the door, that a code was on. Somebody said, "Close the door"—the outside door to the unit, which the Ns with the new pt were holding open . . .

When the new pt was brought in and rolled into his room, the family with him was stopped at unit door, told to stay in waiting room and "we'll call you" with a casual wave of hand, as if this is routine. [No one said a code was on. Patient lying on gurney was wheeled in, went right by the code room and never knew a thing.] [Field Notes]

This is a simple example of protecting the routine from the chaos of a panicking patient or a horrified family; the outsiders never knew that a resuscitation was occurring fifteen feet away. The staff's work was, in their own eyes, routine; their challenge was protecting that routine from outside disruption.

2. *Follow routinization rituals.* The staff's sense of routine is maintained by the protective rituals of hospital life. Under stress, one may use them more and more compulsively, falling back on the old forms to reconvince oneself that order is still present. Frantic prayers in the foxhole are the prototype cases.

Most prominent of such rituals in hospitals are "rounds," the standard ritual for the routine handling of patient disasters in the hospital. "Rounds" is the generic term for almost any organized staff group discussion of patients' conditions. "Walking rounds" refers to a physician walking through the hospital, usually trailed by various residents and interns, going from patient to patient and reviewing their condition. "Grand rounds" are large meetings of the medical staff featuring the presentation of an interesting case, with elaborate discussion and questions, for the purpose of education and review of standard practices. Nursing rounds usually consist of a meeting between the staff for one (outgoing) shift reporting to the staff of the next (incoming) shift on the condition of all patients on the floor. Here the staff collectively explains what has happened and why, bringing every case into the staff's framework of thinking, and systematically enforcing the system's capability for handling medical problems without falling to pieces. In rounds, the staff confirm to each other that things are under control. Once a week, for instance, the Burn Unit at one hospital holds rounds in their conference room with a group of residents, one or two attendings, several nurses, the social workers, dieticians, and physical therapists. The patients here are in terrible shape; one can sometimes hear moans in the hallway outside as patients are taken for walks by the nurses. But rounds continue:

> Macho style of the docs very evident . . . Resident will present a case, then the attendings take rapid-fire shots at what he [the resident] had done: wrong dressing, wrong feeding schedule, failure to note some abnormality in the lab results. Much of the talk was a flurry of physiological jargon, many numbers and abbreviations. The intensity of the presentation, the mercilessness of the grilling, is surprising . . . Focus is on no errors made in situation of extreme pressure—i.e., both in patient treatment and then here in rounds presenting the case. Goal here is to be predictable, *controlled,* nothing left out. [Field Notes]

3. *Use humor to distance yourself.* Keeping outsiders away and following the standard rituals for maintaining normality can help, but sometimes the pathos of hospital life becomes psychologically threatening to staff members. One response is to break down, cry, and run out, but this is what they are trying to avoid; the more common reaction is the sort of black hu-

mor that notoriously characterizes hospitals and armies everywhere. Humor provides an outlet; when physical space is not
available, humor is a way to separate oneself psychologically
from what is happening. It says both that I am not involved
and that this really isn't so important. (In brain surgery, when
parts of that organ are, essentially, vacuumed away, one may
hear comments like "There goes 2d grade, there go the piano
lessons," etc.) With laughter, things seem less consequential,
less of a burden. What has been ghastly can perhaps be made
funny:

> Today they got a 600-gram baby in the Newborn Unit. When
> Ns heard [the baby] was in Delivery, they were praying, "Please
> God let it be under 500 grams"—because that's the definite
> cutoff under which they won't try to save it—but the doc said
> admit it anyway. Ns unhappy.
>
> I came in the unit tonight; N came up to me and said
> brightly, with a big smile, "Have you seen our fetus?" Ns on
> the Newborn Unit have nicknames for some. There's "Fetus,"
> the 600-gram one; "Munchkin"; and "Thrasher," in the corner,
> the one with constant seizures. Grim humor, but common. ["Fe-
> tus" was born at 24 weeks, "Munchkin" at 28.] [Field Notes]

The functions of such humor for medical workers have
been described in a number of classic works of medical sociology. Renée Fox, writing in her book *Experiment Perilous* about
physicians on a metabolic research unit, says, "The members
of the group were especially inclined to make jokes about
events that disturbed them a good deal," and she summarizes
that

> by freeing them from some of the tension to which they were
> subject, enabling them to achieve greater detachment and equi-
> poise, and strengthening their resolve to do something about
> the problems with which they were faced, the grim medical
> humor of the Metabolic Group helped them to come to terms
> with their situation in a useful and professionally acceptable
> way.[3]

3. Renée C. Fox, *Experiment Perilous* (New York: Free Press, 1959; reprint ed.,
Philadelphia: University of Pennsylvania Press, 1974), pp. 80–82.

Fox and other students of hospital culture (notably Rose Coser)[4] have emphasized that humor fills a functional purpose of "tension release," allowing medical workers to get on with the job in the face of trauma; their analyses usually focus on jokes explicitly told in medical settings. This analysis is correct as far as it goes, but in a sense I think it almost "explains away" hospital humor—as if to say that "these people are under a lot of strain, so it's understandable that they tell these gruesome jokes." It suggests, in a functionalist fallacy, that jokes are made because of the strain and that things somehow aren't "really" funny.

But they are. An appreciation of hospital life must recognize that funny things—genuinely funny, even if sometimes simultaneously horrible—do happen. Hospitals are scenes of irony, where good and bad are inseparably blended, where funny things happen, where to analytically excuse laughter as a defense mechanism is simultaneously to deny the human reality, the experience, that even to a nonstressed outsider *this is funny*.[5] The humor isn't found only in contrived jokes but in the scenes one witnesses; laughter can be spontaneous, and it's not always nervous. True, one must usually have a fairly normalized sense of the hospital to laugh here, but laugh one does.

Certainly, the staff make jokes:

In the OR:
"This is his [pt's] 6th time [for a hernia repair]."
"After two, I hear you're officially disabled."
"Oh good, does that mean he gets a special parking place?"
[Field Notes]

In the ICU, two Ns—one male, one female—working on pt.
Nurse 1 (male): "This guy has bowel sounds in his scrotum."
Nurse 2 (female): "In his scrotum?"
Nurse 1: "Yeah, didn't you pick that up?"

4. Rose Laub Coser, "Some Social Functions of Laughter," in Lewis Coser, *The Pleasures of Sociology,* edited and with an introduction and notes by Lewis Coser (New York: New American Library, 1980), pp. 81–97.
5. The genius of Shem's *House of God* is that it accepts this fact and presents it honestly.

> Nurse 2: "I didn't put my stethoscope there!" (Big laughs.)
> [Field Notes]

Sometimes jokes are more elaborate and are obviously derived from the tragedy of the situation:

> In another ICU, staff member taped a stick to the door of the unit, symbolizing (for them) "The Stake," a sign of some form of euthanasia [perhaps the expression sometimes used, "to stake" a patient, derives from the myth that vampires can only be killed by driving a stake through the heart]. Periodically word went around that a resident had just won the "Green Stake Award," meaning that he or she had, for the first time, allowed or helped a patient to die. [Field Notes]
> Some colorful balloons with "Get Well Soon" were delivered to a patient's room. The patient died the following night. Someone on the staff moved the balloons to the door of another patient's room; that patient died! Now the staff has put the balloons at the door of the patient they believe is "most likely to die next." [Field Notes]

But jokes have to be contrived; they are deliberate efforts at humor and so make a good example of efforts to distance oneself, or to make the tragic funny. But the inherent irony of the hospital is better seen in situations that spontaneously provoke laughter. These things are funny in themselves; even an outsider can laugh at them:

> Nurse preparing to wheel a patient into the OR tells him, "Take out your false teeth, take off your glasses . . . ," and continuing, trying to make a joke, "Take off your leg, take out your eyes." The patient said, "Oh, I almost forgot—" and pulled out his [false] eye! [Interview]

Or:

> Lady patient [Geriatric floor] is upset because she called home, there's no answer; she's afraid her husband has died. Sylvia [a nurse] told her he probably just went somewhere for lunch, but patient said he would have called. She's afraid.
> [Later] Sylvia went back in lady's room—she's crying. Husband called! Sylvia happy, smiling, "You should be happy!"

"But," says the old lady, "he called to say he was out burying the dog!"

Sylvia had to leave the room because she was starting to laugh; she and Janie laughing at this at the N's station, saying it's really sad but funny at the same time. [Field Notes]

Or:

In looking at X-rays of a patient's colon, the resident explains to the team a shadow on the film: "Radiology says it could be a tumor, or it might just be stool." Jokes all around about how "helpful" Rays [Radiology] is. [Field Notes]

One needn't be under pressure to find such things funny. People do laugh to ease pressure or to distance oneself. But sometimes the distance comes first: laughter is made possible by the routinization that has gone before.

4. *When things fall apart, keep going.* Sometimes routinization fails: outsiders come into the room and, seeing their dead mother, break down, screaming and wailing; or a longtime, cared-for patient begins irretrievably to "decompensate" and lose blood pressure, sliding quickly to death; or emergency surgery goes bad, the trauma shakes the staff, and there are other patients coming in from the ambulances. Any of these can destroy the staff's sense of "work as usual." In such cases, the typical practice seems to be, remarkably: just keep going. Trauma teams specialize in the psychological strength (or cold-bloodedness, perhaps) to continue working when the world seems to be falling apart. Finally, nurses and physicians are notable for continuing to work even, in the final case, after the patient is for almost all purposes dead, or will be soon.

A resident said to the attending on one floor, discussing a terminal patient: "If we transfuse him, he might get hepatitis."

Another resident: "By the time he gets hepatitis he'll be dead."

Attending: "OK, so let's transfuse." [Field Notes]

Perseverance is a habit; it's also a moral imperative, a way of managing disaster as if it were routine.

In every unit there are nurses known for being good under pressure. These are people who, whatever their other skills (and, typically, their other skills are quite good), are able to maintain their presence of mind in any crisis. Whereas "being organized" is a key quality for nurses in routine situations, staying calm is crucial in emergency situations. Compare two nurses known for remaining calm (Mavis and Anna) to two others who are prone to alarm (Linda and Julie):

> Mavis [in Neonatal ICU] is cited as a good nurse (great starting IVs, e.g.) who doesn't get shook, even in a code, even if her pt is dying, she still keeps doing what you're supposed to do. Linda, by contrast, is real smart, very good technically, but can freak out, start yelling, etc., if things are going badly. [Field Notes]
>
> Julie [in Medical ICU], hurrying around, looks just one step ahead of disaster, can't keep up, etc. Doc says something about the patient in room 1. Julie says, walking past, "He's not mine," keeps going. But Anna, calm, walks in pt's room—pt with oxygen mask, wants something. Anna goes out, calmly, comes back in a minute w/cup of crushed ice, gives pt a spoonful to ease thirst. She *always* seems to be doing that little thing that others "don't have time for"—never flustered and yet seems to get more done than anyone else. [Field Notes, Interview]

But to "keep going" depends not so much on the individual fortitude of nurses such Mavis and Anna, but on the professional and institutional habits of the nursing staff and the hospital. The continuance of care even in the face of obvious failure of efforts is itself a norm. Whatever one's personal disposition, one keeps working; the staff keep working, often when the patient is all but dead, or "dead" but not officially recognized as such:

> Dr. K., walking rounds with four residents, discussing a 30-year-old male patient, HIV-positive, gone totally septic [has bloodstream infection, a deadly problem], no hope at all of recovery—Dr. K. says this is a "100 percent mortality" case; so they decide how to proceed with minimal treatment, at the end of which Dr. K. says brightly, "And if he codes—code him!" [Field Notes]

Coding such a patient is an exercise in technique; there is no hope entailed, no optimism, no idea that he might be saved. There is only the institutional habit which substitutes for hope, which in many cases obviates the staff's pessimism or lack of interest. When standard procedure is followed, courage is unnecessary. It is one thing to be routinely busy, caring for vegetative patients; it happens every day. It is quite another to handle emergency surgery with no time and a life at stake. Sometimes such a case will challenge all the staff's resources—their personal fortitude, their habitualization of procedures, the self-protection offered by an indefatigable sense of humor. To maintain one's composure while under tremendous pressures of time and fatefulness requires all the courage a staff can muster.

One such case was that of emergency surgery on a thirty-five-year-old woman who came to Southwestern Regional hospital in severe abdominal pain; she was diagnosed with a ruptured ectopic pregnancy estimated at sixteen weeks. The case provides us with a dramatic example of the pressure placed on the staff to retain their composure in the face of disaster.

The long description which follows is graphic. The scene was more than bloody; it was grotesque. More than one staff member—including one member of the surgical team itself—left the room during the operation, sickened. Other nurses, even very experienced ones, told me they have never witnessed such a scene and hope never to witness one. I include it here, in some detail, to exemplify both what health professionals face in their work and how, incredibly, some of them can carry on. The description is reconstructed from Field Notes (some written at the time on the inside of a surgical mask, some on sheets of paper carried in a pocket), and from interviews afterward with participants:

Saturday night OR suite; hasn't been busy. Only one case so far, a guy who got beat up with a tire iron (drug deal), finished about 8:30 P.M. It's about 10:00. 2 Ns—the Saturday night staff—sitting around in the conference room, just chatting and waiting for anything that happens.

Call comes over intercom: ruptured tubal (pregnancy) just

came in OR, bringing to the crash room. 35-year-old black woman, very heavy—250 pounds maybe—apparently pregnant for 16 weeks, which means she's been in pain for 10 weeks or more without coming in. Friends brought her to ER screaming in pain. Blood pressure is at "60 over palpable," i.e., the diastolic doesn't even register on the manometer. She's obviously bleeding bad internally, will die fast if not opened up. Ns run to OR and set up fast. I've never seen people work so quickly here, no wasted motion at all. This is full speed *emergency*.

When patient is rolled in, fully conscious, there are more than a dozen staff people in the room, including three gynecological surgery residents, who will operate; all three are women. The surgeons are scrubbed and gowned and stand in a line, back from the table, watching without moving, the one in charge periodically giving orders to the nurses who are setting up. At one point there are twelve separate people working on the patient—IVs going into both arms, anesthesiologist putting mask on pt to gas, nurse inserting a Foley [bladder] catheter, others tying pt's arms to the straightout arms of the table, others scrubbing the huge belly, an incredible scene. The patient is shaking terribly, in pain and fear. Her eyes are bugging out, looking around terribly fast. She's whimpering, groaning as needles go in, crying out softly. No one has time even to speak to her; one nurse briefly leans over and speaks into her ear something like "try not to worry, we're going to take care of you," but there is no time for this. I've never seen anyone so afraid, sweating and crying and the violent shaking.

As soon as they have prepped her—the belly cleansed and covered with Opsite, in a matter of minutes, very, very fast, the anesthesiologist says, "All set?" And someone says "yes," and they gas her. I'm standing right by her head, looking to the head side of the drape which separates her head from her body; the instant that her eyes close, I look to the other side—and the surgeon has already slit her belly open. No hesitation at all, maybe before the patient was out.

What happened next, more extraordinary than the very fast prep, was the opening. Usually in surgery the scalpel makes the skin cut, then slowly scissors are used, snipping piece by piece at muscle, the Bovie cauterizing each blood vessel on the way, very methodical and painstaking. This was nothing like that. It was an entirely different style. They cut fast and deep, sliced her open deep, just chopped through everything, in a—not a panic, but something like a "blitzkrieg," maybe—to get down into the Fallopian tube that had burst and was shooting blood into the abdomen.

When they first got into the abdominal cavity, usually there would be some oozing blood; here as they opened blood splattered out all over the draping on the belly. It was a godawful mess, blood everywhere. They had one surgeon mopping up with gauze sponges, another using a suction pump, a little plastic hose, trying to clean the way. Unbelievable. They got down to the tubes, reaching down and digging around with their hands. And then they found it—suddenly out of this bloody mess down in the abdomen, with the surgeons groping around trying to feel where things were, out of this popped up, right out of the patient and, literally, onto the sheet covering her, the 16-week fetus itself. Immediately one surgeon said mock-cheerfully, "It's a boy!" "God, don't do that," said the scrub tech, turning her head away.

The scrub tech then began to lose it, tears running down her cheeks. Two other people on the team—there were maybe six around the table—said about the same time, nearly together, "Damien!" and "Alien!" recalling recent horror movies, "children of the devil" themes. The fetus lay on the sheet just below the open abdomen for a few moments. The head surgery resident, working, just kept working. The scrub tech should have put the fetus into a specimen tray, but she was falling to pieces fast, crying, and starting to have trouble handing the proper tools to the surgeon, who said something like, "What are you doing?" At this point the circulating nurse, a man, said, "If nobody else will do it," picked up the fetus and put it in a specimen tray, which he then covered with a towel and put aside. He then told another nurse to help him into a gown—he wasn't scrubbed. This violates sterile technique badly, for him to start handling tools, but the scrub tech was becoming a problem. The circulating nurse then quickly gowned and gloved, gently pulled the scrub tech aside and said, "I'll do it." The scrub tech ran out of the room in tears. And the circulating nurse began passing tools to the surgeons himself. It is the circulating nurse's responsibility to handle problems this way, and he did. Another nurse had gone out to scrub properly, and when she came back, maybe ten minutes later, she gowned and gloved and relieved him; so he (the circulating nurse) went back to his regular job of charting the procedure, answering the phone, etc.

By this time, things were under control; the bleeding was stopped, the tube tied off. The other tube was OK and left alone so the pt can get pregnant again. The blood in the abdomen was cleaned up—over 1500 cc's were lost, that's just under a half-gallon of blood. The pt would have died fast if they hadn't gotten in there.

Within two hours after the patient had first rolled in, the room was quiet, only three staff members left, two surgeons and the scrub nurse closing up and talking quietly. Most of the mess—the bloody sponges, the used tools, and all—was gone, cleared away, and all the other staff people, including the chief surgeon, had left. Very calm. The patient, who two hours ago was on the end of a fast terrible death, will be out of the hospital in two days with no permanent damage beyond the loss of one Fallopian tube. [Field Notes, Interviews]

In this situation, we can see two somewhat distinct problems in maintaining the routine order of things: first, the challenge simply in getting the work done; and second, the challenge of upholding the moral order of the hospital.[6] The first issue was resolved by replacing the scrub tech so the operation could continue. The second issue is trickier. The scrub tech's response appeared to be set off not by the horror of what she saw—the bloody fetus—but by the reaction of the assisting surgeon—"It's a boy!" I can only guess that the joke was too much for her. In continuing to work without her, and continuing without noticeable change of demeanor, the surgical team was asserting not only the imperative to protect the operational routine but also, I think, to protect the moral order of emergency surgery as well. That order includes:

1. The job comes first, before personal reactions of fear or disgust.

6. I am indebted to Robert Zussman, who suggested these in his review of the manuscript.

2. Cynicism is an acceptable form of expression if it helps to maintain composure and distance.

3. The medical team is rightfully in charge and above what may be happening in the OR.

4. Preserving life is the central value; others (such as niceties of language or etiquette) fall far behind.

There is clearly a morality here. Just as clearly, it is not the morality of everyday life.

CONCLUSION: THE TRANSFORMATION OF THE MORAL WORLD

1. *The Setting of Limits.* In concluding the second of two chapters on the uses of routinization, I would like to make two final points: first, that every nurse does set limits to what she can tolerate; and second, that routinization entails a transformation of the moral world. In accommodating herself to the radically different world of the hospital, the nurse comes to routinize her experience there, learning the techniques and the people, developing methods for coping with emergencies, training herself to survive disaster and keep working in the midst of appalling tragedy. Quite a few nurses actually enjoy the challenge of pushing themselves to the limits of tolerance, and they seek out jobs that require coolness in the face of stress—emergency room work, ICUs, or helicopter "Life Flight" services. Like the circulating nurse who took over in the OR when the scrub tech fell apart, they rise to the occasion and find their strengths in emergencies; they hold on when others let go. Such nurses live on a thin edge between boredom and chaos: "After a few slow days," says one, "I'm ready for a disaster. I need to be, in a sense, overloaded all the time or I'm not happy." In the words of a floor nurse, such nurses "need their crisis fix" each day. They like the pressure that drives other nurses out of the profession; "The same thing that causes burnout," says the head nurse of one Cardiac Care Unit, "is what I most enjoy."

Still, every nurse, even the most aggressive intensive care nurse, has limits to the sights she can tolerate, to the work she will carry out. For some, relatively minor if disgusting sights are too much. Anderson provides a clear example:

> Some nurses become really upset about bowel movements. They won't empty a bedpan or change a colostomy bag without putting on gloves. Cleaning up after incontinent patients can be messy, especially if the patient has had diarrhea.
>
> It never bothered me to empty bedpans or clean up feces. After all, stool is just breakdown products. It's nothing but what goes into you. What does bother me is watching a patient vomit . . . I have held basins for patients and, while they're vomiting, I'm turning my head and dry-heaving myself.[7]

Here the nurse is rejecting, with her own body, the sights before her. But this is a simple case, one that every mother of a small child has dealt with. In the acute care hospital with seriously ill patients, the challenges to the nurse's eyes and stomach are more severe.

> Geriatric nurse tells of a patient, a fungus had eaten away the whole side of his face, so inside of mouth was exposed, teeth and all, all the way up to one eye. It couldn't be stopped; she had to debride the dead tissue at each stage. [Interview]

Or:

> A nurse now caring for a dying AIDS patient tells me she once cared for a lady with both legs amputated; one was infected, bone sticking out, bloody, smelly, black with necrosis—she had to pick up the stump, clean it, scrub it. Now, as she tells this— sitting outside a dying AIDS patient's room—she grimaces, covers her face with her hands as she describes scrubbing that stump. [Interview]

The nurse, it seems, has implicitly set limits to her own tolerance. When watching a patient vomit, one nurse herself retches; her stomach is saying, "I reject this." Another nurse, telling of cleaning a blackened stump of a leg, hides her face with her hands; her gesture says, "I don't want to see this." The gestures, even more than the nurse's spoken words, point out the limits of tolerance.

7. Peggy Anderson, *Nurse* (New York: Berkeley Books, 1978), p. 32.

These limits are expressed in nurses' preferences for working in, or avoiding, particular services of the hospital. Some Medical [adult] ICU nurses say they could never work with deformed newborns; some neonatal nurses say they couldn't work with quadriplegics; neurosurgical nurses who care for quadriplegics might hate caring for geriatric patients. Almost all nurses refer in interviews to floors or units where they could not work, expressing not just a lack of interest but often a moral distaste for the patients, or their problems, or the work required. In different areas, nurses view different things as personally or morally difficult.

> A nurse on a medical floor said she wouldn't work in the ICU; she wanted to "get rewards from people, not machines." [Interview]
> Why does she like Neuro? The patients can't talk to you, they're out of it usually. [Interview]
> Geriatric nurse says she could never work in Pedi[atrics] because no matter how much you explain, etc., giving a shot or doing something, the kid is still afraid of you—"you're causing pain." She can't deal with that. But "we probably change poo-poo and pee-pee more than everybody else." [Interview]

So almost every nurse has these limits, and this is reflected in the choice to work in one unit and not another. It seems, to speculate here, that nurses almost *need* to say, "I have my limits"; even if I work in a difficult job, I still couldn't do that; *that* would really be tough. Neonatal ICU nurses, handling terribly ill newborns, find their job difficult but believe pediatrics would be impossible; pedi nurses find their task, surprisingly to some outsiders, rather pleasant and their patients easy; geriatric nurses don't mind the mental lapses of their clientele. What appeals to the psychiatric nurse—close personal patient contact—is precisely what the neurosurgical nurse, caring for the physical needs of a comatose automobile wreck victim, most wants to avoid.

In every case the nurse has limits. Her world is different from that of the layperson in its routine, but it has a distinct moral landscape, with a distinction of "tolerable" and "too much." It is as if we all need that contrast to preserve the sense that we are human beings with sensitivities and feelings—the sense that routinization does, after all, have its limits.

So while the "normal" center of the nurse's world has moved from where it was for the rest of us, there is still definitely a center, and deviations from it are still recognized. Throughout this chapter I have given examples of how nurses can adapt to spectacular modifications in what counts as a "routine" day. In the hospital, death is common, suffering is the norm. But nurses who continually deal with death and suffering preserve a sense that even if they are temporarily "dehumanized" (by their own description), still they are sensitive people, not cold-blooded or crassly amoral. Their limits are professionally different than ours, but they have limits nonetheless.

2. *Routinization transforms the moral world.* Routinization entails an implicit decision to modify what counts as normal. In the hospital, what was sacred (handling and inspection of bodies) becomes ordinary; what was unique (the human being with a disease) becomes just another case; what was serious (the death of a pet, the resuscitation of a dying old man) becomes funny; what was grotesque or disgusting (facial fungi, necrotic stumps) becomes a tale to tell over lunch. Instead of tying old people to bed rails, nurses "restrain" them; instead of doping up a crazy lady, they "sedate a confused patient." In becoming a nurse, then, one transforms important elements of one's moral world. The transformation is based on specific learning, as we have seen, but there is more to it than that. Routinization is more than the sum of many specific concrete activities (although it is that); it really does seem, finally, to happen "one day," as the nurses put it. Their "frame" has shifted, to use Erving Goffman's term.[8] What in daily life would be outrageous—a body sliced by a knife, a throat invaded with a metal tube—in the medical context becomes normal, a relatively routine procedure.

This is why so much of conventional debate about medical and nursing ethics is inadequate: the frame shift of routiniza-

8. Erving Goffman, *Frame Analysis: An Essay on the Organization of Experience* (New York: Harper & Row, 1974). I am grateful to Robert Zussman for suggesting this reference.

tion has bracketed out a vast array of moral difficulties. Every-day hospital practice does not present itself as the typical "ethics dilemma" discussed by hospital committees of lawyers and doctors and chaplains; it is not typically discussed in philosophy books, or covered in *Time* magazine articles about young women, victims of car accidents, who have been vegetative for six years. Those cases are dramatic, notable. Many times during my research nurses have asked me if I was meeting with ethics committees, going to official "ethics rounds," or talking with Dr. So-and-So, the renowned "ethics guy" in the hospital. "If you want to know about ethics, you should . . . ," they would say. But behind them, just over their shoulders, would be a young man dying of AIDS whose parents refused to visit him; or an old woman, who when not lost in a drugged stupor would beg to die; or a hopelessly deformed infant who hadn't breathed on her own for four months. Committees only hear of such cases if they become problems, and committees are themselves unusual groups. Hence ethics committees and ethics rounds are a poor site for discovering what typically occurs. This is not to say that nurses aren't aware of the problems under their own noses, but often they don't see them as "ethics problems," and neither do the powers that be, nor the media, nor the academics who talk about such things. The great ethical danger, I think, is not that when faced with an important decision one makes the wrong choice, but rather that one never realizes that one is facing a decision at all.

To an outsider the ordinary work of the hospital is itself morally problematic. The bureaucracy of the hospital poses a problem; the "professionalization" of staff has moral implications; the objectification of patients' bodies matters far more than the official "ethics dilemma" which occasionally pops its head above the surrounding routine. In the normal course of "getting used to" the hospital, nurses and other health care workers become in some measure inured to the profound differences between the hospital and the world beyond it. And if this routine is itself morally problematic, this fact is far more important than whether to continue tube feedings to a patient who for half a decade has been comatose.

Routinization—the acceptance of the hospital as a normal place—happens in the course of things, and often the transition itself is unnoticed ("I can't say exactly when it happened"). Readers of this book may have undergone a kind of routinization experience during their reading, becoming used to the examples, starting to learn a little of the jargon, seeing one or two of the same faces in these pages, beginning to be less shocked by later hospital scenes than by those in the beginning of the chapter. The readers may have, in a sense, forgotten that hospitals are unusual; it really isn't normal for people to do what is being done in the operating room, or to say what people there say. As the shock value of these stories wears off, the change is not in the stories but in readers' attitudes toward them. And it happened somewhere in the reading.

A nurse is, among other things, a person who has undergone such a change. Whether she does right or wrong in her work is not the issue here. We note only that she has become, for good or for ill, part of the hospital itself, and she has done this in a certain style: that of the nurse. Routinization affects physicians, aides, and other hospital workers as well as nurses. But nurses have a special place in this organization, and the particulars of their role are vital for understanding what goes on there. The nurse is the subject of Chapter Three.

THREE

What It Means
to Be a Nurse

So what, then, does it mean to be a nurse?

We have found a huge gap between the nurses' world and ours. For her, the hospital is a normal place, and with routinization even traumatic events that occur there appear normal. What once was a frightful emergency to the novice has become, more and more, just the "same ol' same ol'." The nurse now casually handles naked bodies, measures output of stool, suctions fluid from patients' lungs, passes knives to surgeons, and, just as routinely, cares for the dying. None of this, once she has made the "leap" into a routine, disrupts her daily life or causes her any special concern.

This attitude radically separates nurses and other health workers from the rest of us, and the separation is *morally* relevant, a distance between what nurses and laypersons see as "the right way to behave." Patients are regularly subjected to events no one outside the hospital would willingly undergo. Invasive procedures, humiliating exams, and radical surgery are considered not only acceptable but even in a sense good; the staff rarely gives them a passing thought. Not only is there a shift in what is thought good and what is thought bad; some very serious matters are not much thought about at all. Routinization means that once-crucial issues have been set aside: "These," it declares, "need not concern us."

Of course, routinization of hospital life is not peculiar to nursing. Physicians undergo a similar process, becoming bored with routine physical exams, hurrying through colonoscopies, pelvic exams, and assorted consultations; so too, in varying degrees and in their own activities, orderlies, blood technicians, and respiratory therapists find their work taking on the rhythm of everyday life. Occupational therapists may work every day with children who have cerebral palsy, surgeons quickly get used to removing gall bladders, aides get used to wiping bottoms, and hospital secretaries learn to comfort crying relatives and guide wandering geriatric patients back to their rooms. In all of the health care professions, repeated encounters with messiness, confusion, and tragedy dull the senses a bit, professional jargon softens the hard edges, and jokes become genuinely funny. All hospital workers experience routinization; nursing is not special in this.

But some things *are* special about nursing. The nurse is a particular kind of hospital worker, one with at least three difficult and sometimes contradictory missions. The hospital nurse is expected, and typically expects herself, to be simultaneously (1) a caring individual, (2) a professional, and (3) a relatively subordinate member of the organization. Nurses will argue, even among themselves, just what these directives require, or even that they should exist. (Many nurses will say, for instance, that they should not be subordinates.) Regardless, these three principles tell us who nurses really are and what they really do.

The inherent conflict of these demands makes nursing a prototype case for a dilemma of many workers in an organizational society: I want to do good, but my boss won't let me. The directives conflict: be caring and yet professional, be subordinate and yet responsible, be diffusely accountable for a patient's total well-being and yet oriented to the hospital as an economic employer. Perhaps no other occupation suffers so great a conflict between the practical requirements of the job—and nursing is, rhetoric aside, still fundamentally a job, a paid assignment—and the explicitly moral goals of the profession. Perhaps these are dilemmas of all the "caring" professions (teaching, social work, nursing). Or perhaps they somehow typify predominantly female professions. With more women entering the labor force, with the caring professions growing, and with an increasing proportion of all Americans working under the control of large organizations, increasing numbers of Americans may face conflicts such as those faced by nurses.

In this chapter, these three requirements of the nurse's

role will be examined—the directives of caring, being a professional, and being a subordinate. Then the difficult theoretical
issue of nursing as a "female" profession will be considered.
Finally, I will suggest why nursing ethics should matter to the
rest of us. In nursing, I think, we can see how morally concerned but subordinate people in organizations handle moral
problems in their work.

NURSES CARE FOR PATIENTS

"Care" is the key term in nursing's definition of itself, and
crucially defines what nurses believe is their task. Anytime a
group of nurses talk with an outsider about their work or its
meaning, someone will certainly utter this most positive of
nursing words. Important books about nursing use it in their
titles;[1] job advertisements in nursing journals depict nurses
holding small children, or smiling at an elderly patient, and
promise job applicants to their hospital the unrestricted opportunity truly to "care." Care, some nurses say, distinguishes
nursing from medicine: "Nurses care, doctors cure"; and while
physicians might dispute the moral connotations of that slogan,
few would completely deny its message. "Caring" figures cen-
trally in the stories nurses tell of their own best work experiences. It may be true, as historian Susan Reverby says, that "a
crucial dilemma in contemporary American nursing" is "the
order [to nurses] to care in a society that refuses to value caring,"[2] but among nurses, the willingness to care when that is
difficult is the distinguishing mark of the nurse.

As nurses use the term, "care" seems to include four meanings: face-to-face working with patients, dealing with the patient as a whole person, the comparatively open-ended nature
of the nurse's duties, and the personal commitment of the
nurse to her work. All of these are included in what nurses
mean by "caring." To a moderate degree, "caring" describes

1. For instance, Patricia Benner and Judith Wrubel, *The Primacy of Caring:
Stress and Coping in Health and Illness* (New York: Addison-Wesley Publishing
Co., 1989); or Susan M. Reverby, *Ordered to Care: The Dilemma of American
Nursing, 1850–1945* (New York: Cambridge University Press, 1987).
2. Reverby, *Ordered to Care*, p. 1.

what nurses actually *do;* to a great degree, it describes what nurses believe they *should* do.

1. *Nursing care is hands-on,* a face-to-face encounter with a patient. Unlike in medicine, in nursing there can be no quick review of lab reports, a scribbling of orders, and then a fast exit down the hall. Nurses carry out the scribbled orders, deliver the medications, pass the food trays, monitor the IVs and the ventilators. Nurses give baths, catheterize patients, turn patients who cannot move themselves, clean bedsores, change soiled sheets, and constantly watch patients, writing notes on their patients' progress or deterioration. Close patient contact, with all five senses, is nursing's specialty. ("I could never be a nurse," says one unit clerk. "I couldn't stand all those smells.") Nurses are constantly talking with, listening to, and touching their patients in intimate ways; the prototypical, universal dirty work of nursing is "wiping bottoms." One nurse explains why in her unit nurses no longer wear the classic white uniform:

> It wouldn't stay white very long: there's red blood, feces of various colors, green bile, yellowish mucous, vomit, projectile defecations. [Field Notes]

Physicians visit floors to perform major procedures (inserting tubes into the chest, bronchoscopies); but most of what is said and physically done to patients is said and done by bedside nurses.

The nurse works primarily in a contained space, on one floor or unit; if the patients are very sick, she stays in one or two rooms. She is geographically contained and sharply focused, on this room, this patient, perhaps even this small patch of skin where the veins are "blown" and the intravenous line won't go in. She remains close to this small space, or on the same hallway, for a full shift, at least eight hours and in intensive care areas twelve hours; often she is there for two or even three shifts in a row. With the chronic shortage of nurses she frequently stays and works overtime. I have known a sizable number of nurses, in different hospitals, who worked double and triple shifts—up to twenty-four straight hours—on both floors and in ICUs. One such nurse enjoys double shifts because "I don't have to rush [to finish paperwork] . . . if it isn't done in the first shift, I'll get it done in the evening." So nurses have close contact with their patients over time, hour by hour if not minute by minute, for an extended period of time— "around the clock," they say, and sometimes this is precisely true. This close contact, over time, in a confined space, can give nurses the sense that they know better than anyone else what is happening with their patients; and they may resent any other view:

> Doctor, commenting on geriatric patient: "She looks better today."
> Nurse: "You haven't had to fuck with her all morning."
> Doctor (pause, then tentatively): "She looks better than when she came in." [Field Notes]

No doubt, the "continuity of care" by nurses can be exaggerated by nurses themselves. In fact, with rotating nursing schedules, shifting assignments, the short turnaround time of many nursing tasks, and the constant turnover of nursing personnel, it is not clear that nurses provide continuity at all. Few nurses are actually on the scene "around the clock," and only occasionally is one nurse responsible for the total care of a particular patient. Nevertheless, the geographical restriction of a nurse to one area does enhance her knowledge of the condition of those patients, even when she isn't personally caring for them.

To care for patients, then, first means that one works directly, spatially and temporally, with sick people.

2. *Care means that the patient should be treated not merely as a biological organism* or the site of some disease entity, but as a human being with a life beyond the hospital and a meaning beyond the medical world. Nurses certainly handle the physiological treatment of disease, but they also spend time teaching patients (on dialysis units, e.g., this may be their major task), answering the family's questions, listening to the patient's worries, calling for social service consultations, helping fill out insurance forms, or even, to use a fairly common example, helping an old person find a pair of glasses lost somewhere in the sheets or under the bed. In caring for AIDS patients, nurses often manage negotiations between families and lovers, or among relatives and friends, when families often don't know

the true diagnosis. In all these ways, nurses seem focused on the personal experience of illness:

> [N]ursing appears to be directed to more immediate and experiential goals than medicine: a compassionate response to suffering is more closely identified with nursing than with medicine. Nurses also more often express an interest in disease prevention and health maintenance than physicians. Nurses are less wedded to the physiological theories and diagnostic modes of medical practice. And nursing has a more global and unified science approach to health care.[3]

"Care," then, includes a broad range of the patient's concerns, not just the physical disease itself.

3. *The nurse's duties are open-ended.* Perhaps because of the nurse's sheer physical availability, her job often expands to fill the gaps left by physicians, orderlies, or even families. Some duties are prescribed, but many are not. "To care" for a nurse comes to mean that the nurse will handle problems that arise, whether or not they are part of her official tasks. This occurs for practical reasons. "The nurse," in the words of Anselm Strauss, "comes and stays while others come and go . . . *The role of the nurse is profoundly affected by her obligation to represent continuity of time and place.*"[4] Being on the scene, around the clock, means that nurses are there to integrate the different aspects of hospital work: "Since there's no general agreement about what a nurse is, there are no obvious limits to the job."[5]

Thus the nurse takes on more and more tasks, cleaning up the physical and social messes left by others. When doctors don't explain a diagnosis to the patient, when a unit clerk isn't there to answer the phone, when housekeeping has left a sink unwashed or a floor unmopped, when administration hasn't provided the staff to cover the unit, when chaplains aren't around to listen to a family, when the transportation aide

---

3. Jameton, *Nursing Practice: The Ethical Issues*, p. 256.

4. Anselm Strauss, "The Structure and Ideology of American Nursing: An Interpretation," in Davis, *The Nursing Profession: Five Sociological Essays*, pp. 117, 120; italics in the original.

5. Anderson, *Nurse*, p. 31.

hasn't shown up to take a patient to X-ray—then, often, nurses take over and do these jobs themselves, probably grumbling in the process but realizing that it must be done and that nurses will have to live with the results if they don't:

> Everybody else says: "What do you do as a nurse?" And I say, "I do everything that nobody else wants to do." [Interview]

Nurses might say they do this work *because* they "care"; but here there is no distinction between doing and caring. To care is to *do* the leftover work, to take that responsibility, whether ordered to or not.[6]

4. *Caring requires a personal commitment of the nurse to her work.* It requires a commitment of the nurse herself, as a person, to her work. There is an intertwining of professional skills and personal involvement; in a sense, the involvement is the work, in a way not true of more technical occupations. Nurses would say that some excellent surgeons are horrible human beings; but perhaps it is not theoretically possible to be simultaneously an excellent nurse and a despicable person.[7] The job itself seems to call for decency.

In practice, nursing often elicits a deep personal involvement. In the best cases, nurses give and receive with their patients, first giving of themselves and then receiving, in turn, an unusual intimacy and personal satisfaction from helping another person in his or her most difficult time. Patients can be more open with nurses than with their own families, for a variety of reasons: to spare loved ones the truth of suffering, to maintain the dignity of one's body with a spouse, or to protect children from the reality of their mother's imminent death. The caring professional hears of these things without falling apart, so patients often tell nurses what they wouldn't tell anyone else.

> It's the nurse who's there when the patient is upset and crying, especially on those long, dark nights. It's also the nurse who

6. For further elaboration, see Hughes, *Men and Their Work*, p. 74.

7. "The one-caring, in caring, is present in her acts of caring. Even in physical absence, acts at a distance bear the signs of presence: engrossment in the other, regard, desire for the other's well being." Nel Noddings, *Caring: A Feminine Approach to Ethics and Moral Education* (Berkeley: University of California Press, 1984), p. 19.

develops a day-to-day rapport with the patient. Patients can feel comfortable sharing their physical and emotional pain. There is a lot of intimacy involved; it's the same intimacy found with anyone who is terminal. For some reason, people who are dying tend to lessen their barriers. It's a sad phenomenon that we wait until that time to establish those relationships. But it's a privilege for nurses to work in this area [with AIDS patients and dying pts generally], because in no other type of work are you invited into another's soul.[8]

So the first imperative of nursing is to give care—direct, person-to-person, relatively open-ended care. When nurses tell of their best moments in nursing, they tell of giving such care—not of their technical expertise, or their ability to follow complicated orders without bungling, but of care. This is what nurses identify as the meaningful heart of nursing.

Obviously "caring" is also an ideological term, an idealized way of talking about nursing. It is openly used as a weapon in nurses' conflicts with physicians, to distinguish what nurses do ("care") from what doctors do ("cure"), and to assert the nurse's moral superiority. The more challenging "care" is, the greater the moral prestige of the nurse. So when nurses say they "care," this is more than an empirical description of duties; it is a defense of their own importance.

Nurses don't live up to this high ideal of caring all the time. Not at all. But they do accept it as the ideal, and enjoy achieving it now and then, and talk about it as the noblest mission of nursing. Perhaps this is changing with the increasing emphasis on professionalism, a somewhat different principle; but nursing is still, at its center, about caring.

NURSES ARE PROFESSIONALS

So nurses care—but others care as well. Parents care for their children, lovers for their beloved, children for their pets. For nurses, though, caring is a *job,* an economically rewarded task. And it is a certain *kind* of job, one with high demands for

8. Janet Kraegel and Mary Kachoyeanos, *"Just a Nurse"* (New York: Dell Publishing, 1989), p. 16.

education and responsibility and a claim to a special status, commonly called "professional." The first imperative of nursing is to care; the second imperative of nursing is to behave like a *professional.*

The term "professional" is notoriously ambiguous, both to nurses and to social scientists. For nursing, "professional" is an occupational goal and a term of status, indicating feelings that "our work is important," and "our work takes an advanced degree of training; not just anyone can be a nurse and do nursing tasks." It is a claim to high status. To sociologists, the matter of professionalism is more complicated, and first-rate scholars have spent entire careers exploring it.[9] Here I will try to describe what practicing nurses mean by "being a professional"; I will neither defend nor debunk their claim, nor will I argue whether nursing is "really" a profession. I am trying to understand what it means to be a nurse, and the nurse's own notion of "being a professional" is a major part of that self-image.

Being a professional means (1) doing a job (2) that requires special competence and (3) that deserves special status.

1. *Most basically, a profession is a job*—and a good one at that. The most accurate generalization about nurses is not that they care for patients; it is that they are *paid* to care for patients. For many, ideology aside, this is the primary motivation. Nurses typically have little trouble finding work in America, or almost anywhere in the world. It is easy to move in and out of the nursing workforce, taking time out for raising a family, pursuing other careers, or just taking vacations. The unemployment rate for nurses in the United States is typically close to zero, and nurses' salaries rose significantly during the 1980s in the United States, so that by 1990 their typical starting income was close to $30,000. It is certainly a field open to women, requiring no overcoming of the traditional barriers that have kept women out of medicine or other professions. In a wide

9. Eliot Freidson, *Profession of Medicine: A Study of the Sociology of Applied Knowledge* (New York: Harper & Row, 1970); Andrew Abbott, *The System of Professions: An Essay on the Division of Expert Labor* (Chicago: University of Chicago Press, 1988); Hughes, *Men and Their Work;* Amitai Etzioni, *The Semi-Professions and Their Organization* (New York: Free Press, 1969).

variety of settings—hospital, home health care, school offices, physicians' offices, etc.—a nurse enjoys work options available to very few other employees. She works for a living and probably would not be nursing were it not for the paycheck.

Since nursing is a job, the nurse is frequently required to deal with unpleasant colleagues, uncooperative patients, frustrating bureaucracies, and the routine difficulties of paid work. Even when nurses hate their patients or disapprove of their identities (casualties of gang wars, drug dealers shot in a deal gone bad), or feel that patients are to blame for their own predicament (smokers with emphysema, or alcoholics with gastrointestinal bleeding), they claim to care for them fully. In a sense, I believe, nurses' talk about disliking certain patients reinforces the pride of professionalism. Whoever the patients are, the nurse still goes to work, delivers meal trays, fills out forms, listens to supervisors, delivers medications, and cleans up messes. She can't just walk away, as a volunteer could, or care only for loved ones, as a mother could. Professionalism, then, first means performing the job.

2. Second, *professionalism requires special competence.* Nursing work is often neither simple nor easy; it can be intellectually, emotionally, and physically demanding. So sheer competence is a value, perhaps the central value in nursing.[10] Some people just can't do the work, aren't organized or responsible enough, lack the manual dexterity to insert IVs or give injections, or don't understand the necessary physiology. Nurses can quickly differentiate the good nurses from the bad based on their ability to do the job, finish the assigned tasks, and not make the disastrous mistakes that can so easily happen. They know which nurses can be trusted and which ones can't:

> "If my baby comes in here," said one pregnant neonatal nurse to her colleague, "swear to me that you'll take care of him. I don't want R—— [another nurse] taking care of my kid." [Field Notes]

Professional competence is most challenged in those emergencies when routines break down. Normally, the professional

---

10. Jameton, *Nursing Practice,* chap. 6.

cares for her clients in the form of a "detached concern"[11]—
holding her personal feelings in check while remaining open
to the feelings of the patient. A special effort is required for a
nurse to keep this "professional" detachment when a critically
ill patient, after coming close to recovery, suddenly codes and
dies.

> Right after the code had started, Madge, laughing nervously as
> the team worked on Mrs. B——, said to me, "Oh, God, I'd just
> written her assessment" [saying she was improving].
> After Mrs. B.'s code was over, and they'd declared her dead,
> Madge (who had nursed her for the past week) immediately sat
> at the rolling desk outside the room and wrote notes for at least
> 1/2 hour, very persistently, almost through tears—her face was
> flushed—when people said anything to her, she answered only
> vaguely, kept her head down writing. [Field Notes]

"Being professional" here may mean, as it often does, going into a bathroom to cry, then cleaning up and coming back
out to continue working for the rest of the shift, trying to
act as if nothing happened. "Competence" includes technical
expertise as well as the personal fortitude to maintain that
expertise under pressure.

3. *A professional deserves special status.* A professional, nurses
feel, deserves respect. Nurses typically feel that they deserve
more respect than they receive, from their colleagues (especially physicians) and from laypersons. They are paid for their
work, but good pay is not sufficient.

> No amount of money is worth what you have to do and what
> you have to put up with. That's it: what you have to put up
> with . . . patients throwing full urinals at you, slapping you,
> biting, fighting, swearing. [Interview]

As professionals, nurses feel they deserve an improved status
and better treatment: polite treatment by doctors, the listening
ear of administrators, the respect of outsiders who too often
treat nurses like maids or waitresses.

In trying to be professionals, nurses strive to differentiate

11. Robert K. Merton, *Sociological Ambivalence and Other Essays* (New York:
Free Press, 1976); the concept is discussed in a number of places in the text.

themselves in the public eye from other occupations. A nurse, they emphasize, is *not* a maid, *not* a waitress, *not* a servant.[12] Nurses commonly mention these "antiroles" in talking about their work, to distinguish nursing from those jobs, even if the tasks themselves may sometimes be similar: answering patient call bells, changing sheets, emptying bedpans, helping patients dress or turn over. Nurses do some things maids do. How then does one change sheets "professionally"? The public, they feel, doesn't understand:

> It bothers me, the chronic stupid image of the nurse, the hand-maid-to-the-doctor thing. I don't take well to people who kid-dingly say, "You just empty bedpans all day long." The public has no idea what nursing really is all about. They can see you giving baths, carrying bedpans, taking blood pressures, temper-atures, whatever. And they think that's all nurses do. [Interview]

A major part of nursing's effort to improve its status has come in changing the educational requirements for becoming an R.N. Initially, such requirements were more vocational than academic. From the late nineteenth century until the middle of the twentieth, most nurses were trained by hospitals, often the Catholic hospitals run by religious orders of nuns, and after three years they were awarded a diploma. These nursing students worked as poorly paid apprentices and received, in turn, the skills to go out and practice on their own. The train-ing was rigorous, often notoriously so, and very applied. The nurses received training, the hospitals had cheap labor.[13]

But since the 1960s, many of the hospital schools have closed down, replaced by academic university or community-college programs. With this change, the tone of nursing has changed.

---

12. I once made the mistake, in a lecture to a nurses' association, of comparing nurses' work to that of these other stereotypically female occupations. The audience didn't actually jeer, but they were visibly displeased by the com-parison.

13. Jo Ann Ashley, *Hospitals, Paternalism, and the Role of the Nurse* (New York: Teacher's College Press, 1977). See also Barbara Melosh, *The Physician's Hand: Work Culture and Conflict in American Nursing* (Philadelphia: Temple University Press, 1982); and Reverby, *Ordered to Care*.

Nursing is no longer the calling it once was, says P.W.; the influence of nuns, so pervasive when she was younger, is now fading, being replaced by the university-trained academic model of nursing. [Interview]

The collegiate nurse has come, perhaps unfairly, to represent the ascendance of education, of science, of classroom training, and of the increased social status of higher education. By comparison, the older, hospital-trained nurse represents more traditional values, the more ready subservience to doctors, the hands-on experience, the "school of hard knocks." As can easily be imagined, this split in the profession, and in what counts as a "real" nurse's education, makes a truly unified effort to improve nursing's status difficult. In addition, social class divisions in nursing between the typically middle-class B.S.N. nurses and the more working-class A.A. or diploma nurses are themselves the basis of much contention.[14] Even nurses' caps, which once symbolized a nurse's status, are now considered by most to be outdated and symbolic of lesser prestige; nurses are abandoning the traditional white uniform dress in favor of scrub suits or even civilian clothes.[15]

Many younger nurses see such changes as good; they mark the path to professionalism. Their formal education is longer, their occupational class is higher, their pay is greater, and their expectations for respect and individual initiative have increased. Professionalism is an ideal, but one which, especially through increased education, can improve their social standing.

NURSES ARE SUBORDINATES

Finally, nurses are subordinates in the hospital hierarchy. Not surprisingly, nurses see this feature of nursing less positively

14. "[C]lass divisions within the nursing culture made a feminist politics difficult to achieve," Reverby, *Ordered to Care*, p. 6.

15. The shift in number of registered nurses coming from diploma programs versus associate and baccalaureate (college-based) programs is dramatic: "More than 90 percent of the nurses [practicing in 1984] who graduated before 1960 were graduates of diploma schools . . . During the period 1980 to 1984, only 17 percent of all registered nurse graduates were graduated from a diploma program." *Facts about Nursing 86–87*, p. 21.

than the injunctions toward care and professionalism. Nurses want to care, and they want to be professionals. They don't always want to be subordinates but without doubt they are, and for the most part they accept this as part of their role. The old hospital-based nursing schools actively taught this: "under the dominance of male doctors and administrators, schools of nursing grew; and they were not noted for their development of independent, thoughtful nurses. Students entered nursing schools already expecting that women would defer to men, and, therefore, that nurses would defer to doctors."[16] Nurses' daily work is guided by others: by administrators, some of whom come from nursing; by head nurses who assign them patients; and by physicians, whose detailed orders structure their medical tasks. Nurses arrive at work at an ordered time, on an ordered shift, on specified days. They report at rounds when scheduled, read reports according to custom, answer beepers, fill out charts, and deliver medications as ordered. It is nurses who prepare the patients before procedures and who clean up afterward, changing the sheets, mopping blood, counting sponges, and calming the patients. Nurses may also see themselves as "cleaning up" in a moral sense: "[T]hese second-rank professions explicitly emphasize their role as saviors of both patient and physician from the errors of the latter."[17] The nurse is thus a stage manager for the dramatic stars, limited by the whims of those stars and by the financial and organizational requirements of the owners and managers.

Nurses aren't always directly under the orders of others, of course. In ICUs, nurses frequently make quick decisions on their own, when no physician is available; in dialysis units, it is nurses who teach patients how to dialyze themselves, who write the manuals for patients to use at home, who decide how long dialysis will continue, and who evaluate the patient's tolerance of the side effects. The nurse's subordination, then, is situational: it is almost total in the operating room, where the entire staff is under the command of a surgeon; in long-term nursing home care, by contrast, nurses are in charge. Nurses often supervise other workers, such as aides, orderlies, and thera-

16. Benjamin and Curtis, *Ethics in Nursing*, p. 79.
17. Hughes, *Men and Their Work*, p. 97.

pists of various sorts. And as nurses climb the status hierarchy, other workers fill the lower positions and are subject to the abuse nurses themselves have long known:

> A nurse made a passing comment to L——, a respiratory thera-
> pist (and an older, black woman), about how she, the nurse,
> would have to do some procedure; as a therapist, L. wasn't
> supposed to do it. Over the next ten minutes, L. kept saying
> when spoken to, "Don't talk to me, I'm just a therapist," or "You
> don't want to ask me anything, I'm just a therapist," or "You
> asking me? A *therapist???*" etc. [Field Notes]

If there is a single dominant theme in nurses' complaints about their work, it is the lack of respect they feel, from layper- sons, from coworkers, and especially from physicians. It is nearly universally felt and resented. "The docs never listen to us," they say, "you don't get any recognition from doctors"; doctors don't read the nurse's notes in the patients' chart, don't ask her what she has seen or what she thinks, they don't take her seriously. The daily evidence for this is truly pervasive; I was genuinely surprised at how common the obvious disrespect is. One day I was talking with several staff nurses in a confer- ence room when a young male physician—probably an in- tern—walked in and asked what a drug was for. Immediately, the assistant head nurse explained quickly and in detail. "Oh yeah," said the doctor, "that's right," and walked out. The nurses began to laugh, and one said to the advisor, "You get an A." And doctors also often ignore nurses' opinions:

> Attending not present today, so the Fellow took charge of doc's
> rounds in the ICU. In discussing one patient, a resident asked
> the nurse taking care of this pt if she had anything to add.
> Before the N finished her first sentence, the Fellow was look-
> ing away, visibly uninterested; by the second sentence he had
> started talking with the other intern. [Field Notes]

Sometimes such ignoring of the nurse's view can have seri- ous consequences:

> At Tuesday's conference on Geriatric floor, with residents,
> attending, social workers, etc., all present, Asst HN said repeat-

edly, "You should look at Mr. F.'s foot, it will be a big problem," etc. She didn't seem to make an impression on the docs.

They did nothing about it. Saturday morning, the residents called an emergency surgery consultation because the foot was badly necrosed. Surgeon looked, said had to amputate above the ankle, maybe even above the knee, to check the sepsis. The Asst Head Nurse, who had warned them on Tuesday, was standing off to one side during this discussion, visibly exasperated. [Field Notes]

Even medical students put down nurses in small ways.

In psychiatry unit: during nursing rounds, one nurse reads aloud, written on chart, as doctor's order: "Make sure patient voids [urinates]."

"Who wrote that?"

"Doctor R.'s little med. student." A good laugh about this, as if the nurse would overlook something so obvious. Getting no respect from docs—even future docs—is a source of aggravation and sometime laughs. [Field Notes]

Here, then, may begin a cycle: doctors don't trust nurses; nurses, not trusted even when they are correct, slack off. The mutual lack of respect shows in various ways. Some nurses complain that doctors doing research projects try to recruit nurses as unpaid research assistants—"You're charting this anyway, can't you just keep another copy of it for my data, too?"—and then become angry if the nurse misses six hours of this charting and the data are lost. Generally, nurses' time is considered less valuable, her work less pressing, her opinions less worthy of consideration.

Outside the door of a middle-aged woman patient, with a steady stream of visitors going in, two nurses and the resident are arguing about acidosis and ventilator settings and what Respiratory Therapy should be doing to suction the patient, all in very technical jargon, decreasing this and increasing that. The nurse who takes care of this patient is very angry, with a constant forced smile she puts on in these situations, and repeating, "I don't really want to discuss it anymore," and "It's obvious what we should do. Just sedate her, that's all you need to do." But

the resident isn't sure at all, and the nurses are at the end of
their rope. [The patient died within days.] [Field Notes]

There are, then, pervasive problems in nurses' work relationships with doctors.[18] In part, the difficulty results from
different views of what the nurse's task actually is. To doctors,
the nurses are there to carry out physicians' orders.[19] Indeed,
many doctors (and many nurses) regard nursing as a sort of
"lesser" medicine, with the subordination of nursing dictated
by the shorter period of training.

> Dr. M., explaining why he should make the DNR decisions—
> and why the nurses should not—explains that the difference
> between him and the nurses is "years of training—I have 6 or
> 10, depending on how you count, and they have 2 or 4—I just
> understand things better." [Interview]

Dr. M. here assumes that nursing is essentially the same as
medicine but with less training. He assumes that nurses share
medicine's basic theory of disease (a physiological disturbance
with psychosocial ramifications) and share medicine's ideas
of the goals of treatment. For many physicians, laypersons,
and even nurses, nursing is basically second-tier medicine,
and nursing education consists of watered-down physiology
courses, using textbooks written by physicians, teaching nurses
how to be "the doctor's helper."

In recent years, this position is formulated in a description
of nurses as "physician extenders," a cost-effective substitute
in areas where there aren't enough physicians—a kind of
"Hamburger Helper"[20] who does the same work for less
money. So the nursing viewpoint is not merely subordinated;
indeed, it is often invisible as a distinct approach. Irving Zola
comments aptly on

> the term "physician's extender." It conveys the image of a gross
> medical appendage—a Rube Goldberg invention. In function,

18. The classic article on how the nurse "plays the game" is C. K. Hofling et
al., "An Experimental Study in Nurse-Physician Relationships," *Journal of Nervous and Mental Disorders* 143 (1966), pp. 171–180.

19. Crane, *The Sanctity of Social Life;* Anderson, *Nurse,* pp. 246–248.

20. I borrow the characterization from Gretchen Aumann, R.N.

it implies only an extension of the physician's work—no new alternative to the care so greatly needed in chronic disease. In responsibilities, it tells the patient that anything of importance is to be left to the doctor. And in potentiality, it says to the holder that he/she is in a job with limited mobility and possibility for growth.[21]

Some nurses feel this notion that they simply practice introductory medicine is insulting; and the general public, not knowing what nurses do beyond following the doctor's orders (which is in fact a large part of the nurse's job), unintentionally disparages nursing as a profession all the time:[22]

> I don't know how many times I've heard people say, "Oh, you're so smart, you should have gone to medical school" . . . I wouldn't be a doctor for all the tea in China . . . but, I would just like a little human respect. [Interview]

But many, if not most, staff nurses accept the assumption that medicine is superior and that nursing is simply a lesser form of medicine. They try to enhance their own prestige by a kind of "drift to medicine": by going into the more "medical" areas of nursing, like emergency work, or ICUs; by appropriating the scientific and pathophysiological model of disease; and by getting into the "medical macho" of high technology, invasive procedures, and massive pharmacological interventions, all the while setting aside the lower status "dirty work" of nursing. Although nursing as a profession tries to distance itself from medicine, establishing its own expertise, the typical nurse takes respect where she finds it, from her close association with doctors.[23]

---

21. Irving Zola, *Socio-Medical Inquiries: Recollections, Reflections, and Reconsiderations* (Philadelphia: Temple University Press, 1983), p. 301. See also Zussman, *Intensive Care*, p. 77: "It is by virtue of their technical skills that nurses win the respect of physicians."

22. See also Kraegel and Kachoyeanos, "Just a Nurse," p. 262: "Nursing is a hard job if you have a strong ego. People assume that if you're a nurse, you're doing it because you couldn't be a doctor . . . I know I didn't want to be a doctor . . . yet it still hurts to have people think I wasn't capable of it."

23. Perhaps to the long-term detriment of nursing's effort to independent status. See W. Glasen, in Davis, *The Nursing Profession*, p. 27.

To some extent, nurses' subordination lessened, or at least changed its character, during the period of my research from the late 1970s to the early 1990s. Nurses now more often will openly confront physicians rather than practice subterfuge; they have more ready support from independent nursing schools; perhaps because of the women's movement, nurses are somewhat more likely to expect to be treated with respect, if not really as equals. Still, despite some movement in these directions, nurses remain fundamentally unequal to doctors in their power and status. They are clearly subordinates, much more than their professional leaders or even staff nurses would like to believe. They do important work, and many of them do it with deep personal commitment and a high degree of skill. Yet their subordinate position, more than professionalism and perhaps even more than "caring," is a crucial component of most hospital nursing.

Here we see the dilemma of the nurse's role. On the one hand, she would like to raise her status by both differentiating her work from medicine ("we care, doctors cure") and by claiming to be a professional. On the other hand, by being a necessary member of the medical team she can borrow some of the prestige of medicine. The three components of the nurse's role—caring, professionalism, subordination—all represent in some degree what nurses empirically do and how they interpret what they do. In some ways they are conflicting requirements, fortified by conflicting parties: nursing schools with their admonition to professionalism, administrators with their efforts at controlling nurses, journals with their calls to "care." In some ways, managing these conflicts is inherent in the job of being a nurse.

A FEMALE PROFESSION? A THEORETICAL QUANDARY

So nurses believe they are working in an occupation committed to caring; struggling, against the odds, to gain professional status through the conventional means; and locked into a subordinate position of continually taking orders and doing work that goes unnoticed. Nurses carry out repetitive tasks which, though often highly skilled, are typically undramatic in form and unappreciated by colleagues in surrounding professions and—although this has been changing recently—according to them, financially unrewarded. Not only are they subordinates but their distinctive values and goals, apart from those of medicine, are hardly recognized as existing at all. They feel that their experiences are unrecognized, their complaints unheard;[24] they are, in the current phrase, without a voice. In many respects, then, nursing fits the pattern of many occupations in which women predominate.

Obviously nursing is a "feminine" occupation, both in numbers of practitioners and in style of work. In 1984, 97 percent of the total U.S. population of registered nurses were female; 96.7 percent of employed nurses were women.[25] The 3 percent proportion of men in the profession is only slightly higher than in the past. There's no evidence that this onesidedness in the gender makeup of the profession will change anytime soon. Nursing also exemplifies the style of the historically feminine occupations: an emphasis on caring for others, especially dependents; menial cleaning and housekeeping tasks; relatively low pay and prestige; and an emphasis on helping those (usually men) who are in charge rather than making substantive policy decisions themselves. When I asked nurses the effect of being in a predominantly female profession, they answered with complaints: nurses don't stick together, don't support each other in the presence of superiors, and are too easily intimidated.

But does the "feminine" style of the profession substantially affect the moral judgments of nurses, or the moral character of their work? Initially, it would make logical sense that it does. Ethics are real; they arise in concrete situations, and are lived by real people who are, indeed, male or female. No one has the luxury of a gender-free view of the world, and there is plenty of evidence that the genders see the world differently. Within the world of nursing, people are usually predictably sexed, that is, nurses are overwhelmingly women.

24. Several nurses told me that they had been subjects in numerous retention studies designed to find "what nurses want" but that the administration ignored the findings.

25. *Facts about Nursing 86–87* (New York: American Journal of Nursing Company, 1987), p. 5.

Given that, it would make sense that nurses would view the moral world of the hospital in characteristically female ways.

More specifically, a number of writers have argued that women and men not only have different ideas of right and wrong (e.g., men are more likely to support the use of violence), but that the sexes actually have completely different grounds for moral judgment. They live, that is, in different moral worlds. The standout example of this position is Carol Gilligan's *A Different Voice*. Gilligan argues that while men value independence from others and a reliance on abstract principles in making moral decisions, women put their priorities on maintaining relationships and carrying out an ethic of care in making moral decisions. This argument leads Gilligan to find different conceptions of what is "moral maturity" in the sexes, and finally to argue that women's "different voice" on these matters deserves a recognition and legitimacy that traditional scholars (in particular Gilligan's own teacher, Lawrence Kohlberg) have denied it.[26] Nell Noddings, too, in her book, *Caring: A Feminist Approach to Ethics and Moral Education*,[27] suggests that an ethics based on care for concrete others, not adherence to logically derived abstract principles, is characteristic of women as versus men, and is indeed preferable.

These arguments, though, tend to rely on spoken evidence; they report what women and men *say* rather than what they actually *do*. In the case of nursing, one can watch nurses work and see what they actually do in various situations. And we see that much of their work is determined by others. Embedded in the organization, the nurse typically works on a tight schedule, with a long list of mandated tasks to be done in a limited time, with fairly severe consequences if she fails to complete her work. The tasks, too, must be done according to various defined standards, which are often legally sanctioned—medication doses and delivery routes, standards of care, etc. True, the nurse does have, when there is time (which many say there never is), discretion in talking with patients

26. Carol Gilligan, *A Different Voice* (Cambridge, MA: Harvard University Press, 1982). See also Jean Baker Miller, *Toward a New Psychology of Women*, 2d ed. (Boston: Beacon Press, 1986).

27. Noddings, *Caring*.

and families, or helping other nurses with their work, or teaching. But given the remarkable degree to which her work is dictated in advance and controlled in execution, the wonder is that she can show any ethical decision making at all.

The nature of the job, then, more than an independent "woman's view" or morality, shapes nurses' attitudes. If it is true that "women work with the pervasive sense that what they do does not matter as much as what men do,"[28] this is reinforced, day by day, in their work routines. The job shapes one's view of moral issues as well. For instance, if nurses are more likely than physicians (and I think they are) to support a patient's right to choose or reject treatment, that is because nurses are spending eight to twelve hours each day in close contact with that patient and know how the patient will react to a treatment. The patient's cries will fall on the nurse's ears, the patient's explanations will be given in detail to the nurse. The nurse is the one who will see the family agonizing over a decision to let Dad die, and the nurse will be in the room when he finally passes on. One need not be an especially "caring" individual to demonstrate the objective care that a nurse does when giving a bed bath, or conscientiously debriding a wound. (How does one express "masculinity" or "femininity" in one's nursing care?)[29] Whether the nurse is male or female doesn't change any of this.

In past years nursing was probably more deliberately feminine than it is now. Since women were excluded from most other occupations, and certainly from higher-paying occupations, nursing was an enclave in which they could be employed at tasks (usually private-duty nursing) that cost little and simultaneously reinforced conventional notions of female servitude and personal care. Women were a population that could be subordinate without being socially distant (unlike other servants).[30]

If nurses' moral views reflect their position in the hospital

28. Miller, *Toward a New Psychology of Women*, p. 76.

29. See Christine Williams, *Gender Differences at Work* (Berkeley: University of California Press, 1989), chap. 4 for examples of male nurses explaining the "masculine" way to be a nurse.

30. Suggested by Robert Zussman.

and the nature of their work rather than their gender and the female ethics of their profession, then gender becomes secondary. In radical form, this structural interpretation says that even if all nurses were men and all doctors women, the current system would impel them to act as nurses and doctors now act. Many rank-and-file nurses do, in fact, hold an inchoate version of this view, and so

> nurses have often rejected liberal feminism, not just out of their oppression or some kind of "false consciousness" but because of some deep understanding of the limited promise of equality and autonomy in a healthcare system they see as flawed and harmful.[31]

As things now stand, the structural thesis is hard to test, because of the multicollinearity problem: we cannot distinguish the effect of gender (female) from occupation (nursing) because the two are so highly correlated. There are few men in nursing, they are a highly self-selected group, and they are clustered in a few areas (ICUs, ORs). As far as we know, men in nursing are in fact treated better than comparable women; but we are comparing unconventional men with women who in many respects are quite conventional. It may be, as Rosabeth Kanter suggests,[32] that given the same situation men and women will react more or less the same way; if nurses were all men, perhaps those men would all be caring, concerned with relationships, and interested in the patient as a whole person.

Still, nurses *aren't* all men. The vast majority of nurses are women, and that is no accident. Whatever the utopian possibilities, however difficult it is to analytically distinguish the impact of gender from that of other social structures, the facts are fairly straightforward: nurses are mostly women, doing tasks that are traditionally women's tasks. At the same time, only a few men go into nursing, and then for stated reasons that do not violate the standard gender roles. The best source on the gendered position of men in nursing is Williams: "There are

31. Reverby, *Ordered to Care*, p. 207.
32. Rosabeth Moss Kanter, *Men and Women of the Corporation* (New York: Basic Books, 1977).

few men in nursing because *men do not want to be nurses,* and those who are express strong ambivalence toward their chosen profession. The male nurses I spoke to went to great lengths to distinguish what they do from the traditional conception of nursing tasks."[33] Large numbers of women, in our society, choose to become nurses, while very few men so choose; and the job (as currently defined) calls for those behaviors and attitudes currently seen as "feminine." The structure of the work reinforces and supports the going conceptions of femininity in the larger society, and this is not lost on people choosing (or not) a career in nursing. It may be theoretically plausible to suggest, as Kanter would, that the structure of the work is decisive; but jobs do not exist in the abstract, apart from the capabilities and habits of the people who perform them. The "caring" nature of nursing, the undervaluing of that kind of work, and the assignment of such work to women tell us less about a particular job or hospital than about the position of women in American society.

So nursing is a female occupation, not essentialistically but empirically. That fact, along with the other particulars we've discussed of the nurse's role, shapes the nurse's view of moral issues in the hospital.

THE NURSE'S ROLE: IMPLICATIONS FOR ETHICS

This chapter has explored in some detail what it means to be a nurse. We have already seen that nurses treat their work in the hospital routinely and experience the hospital as a relatively normal place. Nurses understand their work as falling under the sometimes conflicting imperatives of caring for patients, behaving as professionals, and working as subordinates in the hospital organization. These imperatives are simultaneously *prescriptive*—saying what nurses should do—and somewhat *descriptive*—that is, actually reflecting what nurses in fact do. Nursing is basically a female occupation, with low visibility of its work and moderate prestige accorded to it. All of these components of the nursing role are suffused with moral impli-

33. Williams, *Gender Differences at Work*, p. 90. Italics in the original.

cations: they carry moral judgments about who the nurse is and how she should do her work.

That role has implications for the ethics of nurses and for the rest of us. The nurse's position is not so unusual. Many Americans work in the "helping professions," broadly defined, and many more would characterize their work as serving others. While most do not consider themselves professionals, they do take their work seriously. And a growing number of workers are female. The ethical challenges of nurses may suggest the ethical challenges of any caring but subordinate person working in a large organization today. In trying to understand the ethics of nursing, then, we can begin to understand the ethical problems of the rest of us as well.

For this new variant of ethical analysis, several steps are required:

1. *Rediscovering the unappreciated.* Probably the most frequent question I am asked about my research is "Why are you studying nurses?" or even "Why do you care about nurses?" Most people don't care about nurses and, not surprisingly, don't understand the significance of their work. Much of nursing is invisible—to doctors, to patients, and to the layperson. What is noticed—baths, turning patients, routine monitoring—is seen as unimportant, except by patients: "A patient complains about not getting a box of tissues. That may seem unimportant. Yet if the person is lying there with his nose running and he can't get up, that box of tissues becomes monumental."[34] Naturally enough, nurses resent this lack of appreciation; a popular recent book on nursing, by a pair of nurses, is titled, with quotation marks and all, *"Just a Nurse."*[35]

Even when doing recognizably important work, as in the ICUs or operating rooms, nurses are regarded as skilled helpers to the doctors, adjuncts to the people doing the "real" work. It's easy, when watching surgery, to be drawn to the center of the action, where the surgeon is cutting, and away from the nurses arrayed around that center, or walking in the background. On rounds, physicians do the talking while nurses stand by holding charts or quietly attending to some task. With

34. Anderson, *Nurse*, p. 106.
35. Kraegel and Kachoyeanos, *"Just a Nurse."*

physicians holding the dramatic center stage of medical work, nurses become stagehands, secondary figures. The physician's work is valued; nurses' work is valued only as it mimics the physicians: "The most valued forms of competence currently tend to reflect scientific and technological interests—what people consider intellectually difficult, exciting, and challenging—rather than what is most directly related to patient good or to public health."[36] To rediscover their own work and see what they do—to put them, for a moment at least, at the center of their own world—is a first step to understanding who nurses are.

The recovery of unappreciated work is especially relevant when analyzing women's work. As Miller puts it, "All of these things, the things women are allowed to do, are in a significant way removed from the life of one's time. Women's place is outside the ongoing action. To nurse the old, the sick, and the disabled is taking care of those who are temporarily or permanently retired; raising children is an involvement with those who are not yet in the main action. Women even take care of those who are in the main action during the hours of the day when they are out of action—that is, they provide care and comfort to the tired man when he comes home at night. Women's other role, the biological production of the next generation, is deemed essential, but it also positions them effectively outside the action of their own generation. This is one of the circumstances that women refer to when they say they feel they have lost touch with 'the real world.' "[37] But perhaps theirs is the real world, and it is the observers who have lost touch.

2. *Finding an appropriate ethics for nursing.* Nursing ethics is hardly a recognized field of inquiry, even for academics. Books on nursing ethics typically borrow the principles of medical ethics and apply them to nursing situations, with little recognition that the nurse's situation is profoundly different than that of the doctor. Doctors often make critical decisions with little outside help. The prototype medical ethics scenario involves a dramatic case, choices of heroic intervention, a situation of

36. Jameton, *Nursing Practice,* p. 85.
37. Miller, *Toward a New Psychology of Women,* p. 75.

crisis: and now the doctor must choose. Medical ethics is thus characterized by dilemmas in which the lone individual must decide the right thing to do. Philosophical medical ethics largely assumes this freedom of the practitioner to choose; the ethical problem lies in deciding what choice is morally right. But in nursing, the problems are frequently those over which nurses have no control; they are not dilemmas, in the sense of an individual's quandary, at all, and the language of "ethical dilemmas" hardly works for a profession whose work is so determined by the choices of other, more powerful, actors. For doctors, the dilemma may be, "Do we save this baby?" For nurses, the problem is, "How can I care for this baby who is needlessly suffering?" The doctor often *decides;* the nurse more often then *does.*

Since nursing ethics is usually written as a variant of medical ethics, medical hegemony in health care is perpetuated; the distinctive voice of nursing is lost; and the distinctive moral situation of the nurse is lost.

3. *A distinctive ethical analysis is required.* If we are truly to recognize the position of the nurse and see that nursing is not merely a branch of medicine, then a different sort of ethical analysis is required. Medical ethics deals with dilemmas faced by relatively powerful people, but nursing ethics needs to consider the distress suffered by much less powerful people—in this case, the nurses. While trying to do good, nurses are embedded in an organization, responsible for some people and ordered by others. Nurses are enjoined to care for the patient, to be concerned with the patient as a person, and to be professionally responsible. At the same time, devoutly prolife nurses may be asked to help with abortions, to let deformed infants die, to disconnect ventilators from terminal cancer patients. In each of these cases, they may feel the decision is morally wrong. Nurses often must carry out policies they deplore, orders they believe wrong, and treatments they believe cruel. They have little time to consider a range of options, little power to change current routines, and almost no freedom to leave the situation.

Nursing ethics, then, is the ethics of powerless people; the ethics of witnesses, not decision makers; the ethics of implementers, not choosers; the ethics of those whose work goes unnoticed. Perhaps, too, as its practitioners are predominantly women, it is the ethics of more personal relationships: "In particular, it is well known that many women—perhaps most women—do not approach moral problems as problems of principle, reasoning, and judgement."[38] Nursing ethics is the ethics of most of us: not in charge; carrying out the commands of others; trying, within imposed limits, to do the job. There is no special virtue in this. Much of the nursing literature suffers from an exaggerated idealism, and many nurses will in effect say, "I would do things differently if I were in charge." But they aren't in charge, and if they were, experience shows us, they probably would do things the way the people in charge do. Simply being a nurse does not guarantee righteousness. As Zussman says, "[T]hey are more concerned than physicians with comfort and emotional adjustments to illness, less concerned with cure. But this perspective does not make nurses angels of mercy."[39]

In summary, we have seen that nursing has a distinctive moral core—a set of directives that nurses accept as their own, even when they fall short of those standards. The distinctive role of nursing entails a combination of care, professionalism, and a subordinate position, and the style of the profession is obviously female. In many ways, the ethics of nursing points to a broader ethics of organizational life. In understanding nursing, we may better understand the moral position of other organizational subordinates.

Nursing has its own legendary figure who exemplifies best what the profession should, and can, be: Florence Nightingale. The Nightingale legend is strong in nursing, and she stands alone, perhaps more so than the dominant figure of any other occupation. And Nightingale is clearly a nursing heroine. She is not remembered for her scientific contributions (which were significant), or for her contributions to technique. She, instead, is the prototype heroine of organizational underdogs. Nightingale is revered by nurses (she is always mentioned at contemporary nursing conferences) as a strong woman who cut through the organizational red tape to get what her patients needed. "Nobody screwed with her," says one nurse. Nightingale saw

38. Noddings, *Caring*, p. 28.
39. Zussman, *Intensive Care*, pp. 71–72.

problems clearly and then forced the system to respond to her. "She wasn't wimpy about it." It is her moral strength, her character and perseverance in the face of bureaucratic authority, that nurses today respect and hope for in themselves. By successfully fighting the recalcitrant British Army organization in which she worked, Nightingale became a legendary model for nurses. This is appropriate, for it is the hospital organization, as will be shown in Chapter Four, that creates many of the nurse's ethical difficulties.

FOUR

How the Organization Creates Ethical Problems

The hospital as an organization is not merely the setting for moral crises; the hospital's organizational form actively generates such crises. Against a background of routine, structural rifts in the hospital organization—especially those between different occupational groups—emerge as "ethical" differences. When different interest groups collide, and as arguments erupt over work and how it is to be done, these arguments frequently take on a moral tone and become framed as "ethical debates." And as the autonomy of physicians diminishes, there is an increase in these intergroup conflicts, and hence a rise of such politicized "ethical problems."

Thus far, we have mainly examined the nurse's moral *routine*, not her moral *problems*. We found that the hospital has its own unquestioned order; the nurse plays her role within that order. Much there is taken for granted: patients come and go (or die), but the staff goes on, in a daily round of repeated events. The nurse's place in those events is shaped by the nursing imperatives of care, professionalism, and subordination to the administrators and physicians in charge. She lives in a relatively unstudied flow of standard operating procedures.

Sometimes, though, this routine is broken; sometimes the moral taken-for-grantedness of the nurse's world is challenged. Problems arise, issues of right and wrong that cannot be covered by the usual assumptions. These problems strike at the heart of one's identity; they raise questions: "Who am I?" and "What sort of person will I be?" Some such issues become visible and consciously thought about, and nurses come to see them as ethical problems and try to discuss them in terms of a moral code. In this chapter, I will show how these "ethical problems" arise for nurses, and then I will outline a theory of what ethical conflict is and where it occurs. These are fundamental issues for the sociology of moral life.

TWO EMPIRICAL OBSERVATIONS

Two empirical observations will begin our sociological investigation of nursing ethics: first, that nursing's ethical problems are systematic; and second, that they usually involve practical difficulties, not private dilemmas.

1. *Nursing's ethical problems are systematic.* What nurses see as ethical problems arise in predictable settings, over and over again; they are not random events. It's not as if one nurse in an ICU has a problem, then another nurse over in the ER has a different problem, and these are more or less isolated incidents. The same problems recur time and again, in various settings.

This has a specifically sociological implication, which C. Wright Mills once expressed with regard to another social problem:

> When, in a city of 100,000, only one man is unemployed, that is his personal trouble, and for its relief we properly look to the character of the man, his skills, and his immediate opportunities. But when in a nation of 50 million employees, 15 million men are unemployed, that is an [public] issue, and we may not hope to find its solution within the range of opportunities open to any one individual.[1]

When problems are systematic and widespread, they transcend the individual motivations of actors; they instead reveal structural features of the setting. Somehow, one can assume, features of the organization or the work create those problems. Remove a nurse with an ethical problem from the hospital, replace her, and her replacement will encounter the same problem. The problem is not of the person but of the system.

2. *Nurses face practical problems, not individual dilemmas.* The

---

1. C. Wright Mills, *The Sociological Imagination* (New York: Oxford University Press, 1959), p. 9.

ethical difficulties nurses encounter frequently involve the practical problem of accomplishing some task over the opposition of other people: a recalcitrant physician, a family that doesn't understand, administrators who must meet budgets.

Nurses often say, "I *know* what ought to be done, but I can't get it done." Nurses, I think, often have clear ideas of what they believe is right but lack the power to do it over the objections of others. This is the source of the nurse's difficulty, which Jameton, probably the finest observer of these matters in nursing, calls "moral distress":

> Moral distress arises when one knows the right thing to do, but institutional constraints make it nearly impossible to pursue the right course of action.[2]

This lies in dramatic contrast with the traditional academic image of medical ethics. In that view, a lone practitioner (typically a physician) faces a difficult moral decision, a "dilemma." Two conflicting principles battle within his (traditionally "his") mind; he stands alone, unsure of how to decide, wrestling with his own conscience—and, clearly, with the power to decide and make the decision stick. Medical ethics as a discipline has come to his aid, providing articulated philosophical principles on which to act and logics by which to apply the principles.

The language of dilemmas individualizes ethics, making morality a personal issue. The individual is advised to get more education, to change her thinking, to clarify her principles. "Dilemma" refers to an ethical difficulty as something to be solved in the mind of the professional person, an internal balance of positions. The troubled person is said to "be conflicted," as if in a fight with herself.

This neatly avoids the possibility that she has a conflict with someone else. Talk of "ethical dilemmas" diverts attention from the structural conditions that have produced the problem in the first place. This is naturally in the interest of the status quo and is relatively unthreatening to powerful interests within the hospital. This is why so many hospitals can readily accept an "ethics committee" and its debates about ethical issues. Ini-

2. Jameton, *Nursing Practice*, p. 6.

tially, some powerful hospital staff may feel threatened, but the threat is contained by framing issues as "difficult dilemmas" rather than seeing them as symptoms of the structural flaws of the health care system. At the beginning of my research in one hospital, I was repeatedly told by friendly informants not to speak publicly (in seminars, e.g.) about what they all agreed was the *obvious* key to nursing's ethical problems, namely, the organization of the hospital and the health system. "Talk about psychology, not organization," one said. They worried that if I spoke of organizational problems, administrators would swiftly shut down my project.

If ethical problems are not dilemmas, then what are they? For the most part, I will suggest, they are symptoms of occupational group conflicts in the hospital, in which moral arguments are weapons in a fight, usually decided in favor of the greater power. Ethics committees, in turn, are useful not as objective arbiters but as anticipated allies in those fights. Problems are not so much dilemmas of conscience but practical problems dumped on nurses from other units, other institutions, and from the society at large. Debates rage, not within one's own mind but between nursing and administration, nursing and medicine, nursing and society. In the complex hospital organization embedded in a complex society, nursing finds itself at the intersection of competing occupational groups and moral ideologies, and this competition is the source of its ethical problems. Each day nurses juggle the orders of physicians, the needs of patients, the demands of families, the rules of the law, the bureaucracy of the hospital, and their own physical and emotional limits. The conflict of these are expressed as "ethical problems in nursing."

To be sure, there are genuine dilemmas in nursing practice. Imagine that a man suffered a heart attack and is now resting in the Cardiac Care Unit. During his stay, his sister is killed in an automobile accident. When he asks for his sister, should the patient be told the truth—his evident right as a family member—or should he be deceived, and thus perhaps protected from another, probably fatal, heart attack? This is a true dilemma, the kind that nurses occasionally face. Or sometimes a nurse must choose between her own multiple goals, for instance, between caring for the patient and being professionally loyal to a colleague who has made an unintentional mistake.

But in nursing, the old model of ethical dilemmas is becoming obsolete; the diffusion of responsibility makes true dilemmas less and less common. Instead, ethical dilemmas are the moral outcroppings of differences between relatively powerful groups. Ethical problems are no longer the heavy burden of the lone practitioner, such as the traditional physician. There are too many other parties involved: nurses, administrators, families, lawyers. Where power is concentrated and decisions are made by a single person, we find dilemmas. But as a multiplicity of constituencies invade the hospital, then, increasingly, ethical issues entail conflicts between constituencies. In a sense, as everyone in the hospital becomes a subordinate to someone else, then moral problems are externalized and become practical, debatable issues of politics. Even for physicians, ethical problems are now manifestations of conflicts with patients, families, or regulators of some sort.[3] Ethics in the traditional sense of a code for the autonomous individual is becoming outdated; in the increasingly fragmented world of American health care, ethics has been replaced by a (heavily moralized) politics.

A STRUCTURAL THEORY OF ETHICAL PROBLEMS IN ORGANIZATIONS

I propose here a series of basic principles about the emergence of moral issues in organizational settings. These principles don't pretend to explain the emergence of all ethical problems in organizations, but they do, I believe, cover the majority of them. They do so by answering some basic sociological questions: What do ethical issues mean for the people involved, and where do they arise?

1. *Ethical problems reflect the conflict of powerful interest groups.* This is the fundamental principle; the following four essentially elaborate on it. For the most part, ethical problems in organizations do not spring full-blown from the independent

3. Robert Zussman suggested this to me.

mind of a single practitioner, struggling with her lone conscience. They tend, rather, to be specific manifestations of well-articulated disputes between interest groups—typically, between rival professions or constituencies. Consider the common argument between nurses and doctors over whether to halt aggressive treatment of a terminally ill patient. Physicians tend, for a variety of reasons, to lean toward aggressive treatment, perhaps from fear of malpractice suits, belief in the efficacy of medicine, responsibility to save lives, or even a relative ignorance of the patient's suffering. The physician's reluctance to stop treatment conflicts with the nurse's (work-imposed) frustration at dealing, hour after hour, with a patient who isn't progressing and who is begging to be let alone. Nurses thus may lean toward discontinuance of treatment, perhaps from frustration, or pressure from patients or families, or a sense of futility. The situation represents an ethical issue for both parties, but it represents as well a structured conflict of worldviews of the two professions.[4] And since the physicians have the power to make the final decision (although this power can be subverted—see Chapter Six), distraught nurses may call on the hospital's ethics committee, not for an objective appraisal of the situation but for moral support in a professional conflict.

> The Surgical ICU nurses will call for ethics consult tomorrow on "big belly" pt—guy who's septic because of surgical infection, going to die. (They want to let him go.) Docs won't like this. That's how ethics is here—no dilemma, but dispute. [Field Notes]

2. *Fundamental conflicts between groups become labeled as moral conflicts.* What could be described as political arguments or turf battles are translated into moral terms and become "ethical problems." To use the previous example, the nurses will claim that physicians who persist with aggressive treatment are not truly caring for the patient (a basic function of nursing) and that this is immoral, simply wrong, morally wrong. Physicians

---

4. See Renée R. Anspach, *Deciding Who Lives: Fateful Choices in the Intensive Care Nursery* (Berkeley: University of California Press, 1993), for discussions of this.

will respond that the doctor's duty is to save the patient's life; it is all too easy—especially for those nurses doing the dirty work—just to say, "Leave him alone, just let him die." The physician is professionally committed to protecting lives, even terribly damaged ones. This commitment is no mere technical judgment; it strikes at the heart of what it means to be a doctor. So nurses and doctors approach the patient with significantly different goals, and these are described in moral terms.

These two different positions have been fully articulated by well-educated spokespersons for the two professions. Indeed, perhaps it is only with the rise of a profession's intellectuals, or at least articulate speakers, within an occupational group that the group's professional goals become clarified and related so clearly to basic human needs as to become ethical principles.

3. *Ethical issues reflect conflicts of groups' moral agendas.* Being a professional implies, as discussed in Chapter Three, that one personally identifies with one's work; the profession's goals become one's own goals. Nurses want to care for patients, and physicians want to cure patients. Both do so as a committed statement of their own personhood.

So ethical issues often reflect a clash between the competing professional moral agendas. Physicians, morally committed to saving lives, resent interference with that goal. Administrators, morally committed to providing equitable care to patients from all circumstances, are irritated at excessive spending on experimental work. Nurses, morally committed to an integrated caring for patient and family, are upset by the hospital's brusque treatment of relatives. Such tactical disagreements can easily become major conflicts of moral positions in the fragmented but heavily moralized ambiance of the hospital:

> [Nonprofit institutions] have a greater propensity for internal conflict than businesses precisely because everybody is committed to a good cause. Disagreement isn't just a matter of your opinion versus mine; it is your good faith versus mine.[5]

4. *When group statuses shift, ethical problems increase.* As nursing's status has risen, ethical conflicts with other occupational

5. Peter Drucker, *Managing the Nonprofit Organization* (New York: Harper Collins Publishers, 1990), p. 125.

groups have increased. In former years, when nurses were unambiguously subordinate to administration, they faced one major decision: Do I become a nurse? Once the job was accepted, other questions of ethics were more or less resolved. "That's not my decision," was the appropriate response. The physician's moral preeminence was unquestioned; moral issues were taken as matters of professional (medical) expertise. But as nurses have taken on more responsibility, they have come to challenge medical dominance; they have come to feel that they must answer ethical questions for themselves. Indeed, "professionalization" in part describes a shift from a technical to a moral orientation to one's work. As power goes up, so does responsibility. Hence the increase of ethical conflicts.

This trend is accelerated by nursing's increasingly articulate voice. The growth of university departments of nursing, independent of particular hospital settings, has created sizable cadres of academically sophisticated nursing professors. These nursing professors have the time to devote to speaking and writing about nursing, and have the intellectual abilities to promulgate clear, detailed philosophies of the goals and means of nursing itself, apart from those of medicine or the health care establishment. Most staff nurses "in the trenches" of the hospital don't care about academic nursing or the profession at large (". . . only 21 percent of the currently employed registered nurses belong to the American Nurses' Association; this suggests a low interest in professional organization among the rank and file"),[6] it is true. But university nursing schools give the profession an independent base, and their strong independent voice gives nurses an ally in their efforts to make their point of view heard.

The improved status and professionalization of nursing has occurred simultaneously with several other historical developments, which together make nursing more influential. (1) First, there was the public debunking of medicine and the rise of public discussions of medical ethics. (2) Then there was the feminist movement, with awareness of the relative silence of women, and women's increasing awareness that apparently personal problems are often really symptoms of political ineq-

6. Benjamin and Curtis, *Ethics in Nursing*, p. 114.

uities. (3) Finally, we have the chronic short supply of nurses, which makes their occupational security considerably greater than it was in the old days of hospital nursing schools when student nurses were exploited as cheap labor. In short, nurses can now get jobs almost anywhere, and they have developed a voice—stronger in nursing schools, weaker in hospitals—to make their concerns heard. Hence, the growth of "ethical problems in nursing."

5. *Ethical problems change over time.* In just ten years, from 1980 to 1990, there were dramatic changes affecting nursing ethics. The emergence of the AIDS epidemic posed questions of the distribution of scarce resources, the management of severe family disruptions, and the handling of young, terminally ill patients in large numbers. The increased visibility of and efforts at cost control by insurance companies shifted power in health care. DNR ("Do Not Resuscitate") decisions were routinized in procedures required for accreditation of all U.S. hospitals by 1988, so that decisions to terminate treatment were handled by formal procedures instead of ad hoc decision making or medical custom.[7] All of these meant new ethical concerns for nurses.

Nursing has also seen changes in the organization of nursing care. Since World War II and its accompanying shortage of nurses, the most common organization of work has been "team nursing," in which nurses divide up the necessary tasks for a unit of patients among themselves. One nurse gives all the baths, another takes blood pressures, still another passes all the medications. This system efficiently uses the auxiliary staff—practical nurses and aides—to perform the lower-skilled tasks and saves the skilled RNs for more complicated procedures. Each nurse then sees many patients but has only a tenuous connection with any one of them. In recent years some hospitals have moved to "primary nursing," in which each patient has a single nurse, and each nurse is assigned a small number of patients. This "primary nurse" organizes all the care for each of her patients, and knowing patients and families better she may be more likely to feel responsible for

---

7. These policies are those of the Joint Commission on Accreditation of Health Care Organizations.

the patient's well-being. Thus she may be more ready to argue with the physicians or others on what care is being ordered. When the organization of work changes, so too do the ethical conflicts.

These five principles form the heart of my argument. The remainder of this chapter presents a series of demonstrative examples. I don't suggest that the dynamic of group conflicts accounts for all of nursing's moral issues, but it may well explain the majority. When power relationships are stable and unchallenged, there will be few ethical crises; the answers are routinized, the decisions are made by clear authorities, and subordinates do their jobs and keep their mouths and minds shut. But when the authorities become challengeable, when new constituencies come into being, when new occupational groups begin to define and defend their own turf, then the moral agendas of these various groups come into conflict. The resulting quarrels are (correctly) seen as moral conflicts, framed in the formal terms of ethical debate. Such debates, I suggest, will only arise when there are speakers to deliver them, and with a voice strong and clear enough to be heard.

SOME EXAMPLES OF GROUP CONFLICT AS "ETHICAL ISSUE"

The pure "ideal type," in Weber's phrase,[8] of an ethical conflict would involve two professional groups with competing moral agendas. Nonprofit organizations with multiple constituencies and strong moral components (e.g., Christian colleges, nonprofit hospitals, psychiatric social service agencies) might be the most fertile field for this kind of eruption. Variations could involve the clash of any occupational groups with moral commitments, or even with latent moral positions on some issues, probably derived from their own work situations. In practice, such conflicts will often be multisided, with different parties holding different positions, adopting shifting alliances depending on the particular problem at hand. In hospitals, administrators may find physicians to be a scarce resource, and

8. Max Weber, *The Theory of Social and Economic Organization* (New York: Oxford University Press, 1947), p. 92.

thus ally themselves with medicine against the interest of nurses, who are less organized and perhaps less accustomed to asserting themselves. Or administrators who come from nursing may sympathize with the nurses' point of view and find themselves locked in battles with doctors, or families, or even other administrators. In each case, though, their moral positions will derive mainly from the ideologized position of the major occupational groups in the organization.

In each of the following examples, nursing stands on one side of the conflict. I will begin with fairly simple two-sided conflicts and gradually move to the more complex, multisided situations, and even to the widest circles in which nursing finds itself at odds with a vaguely defined "society." Throughout, the presentation will tend to be from the viewpoint of nurses.

1. *Nurses versus doctors.* The simplest case of moral conflict for nurses occurs vis-à-vis doctors—"physicians," as they are often called by nurses, in a pointed avoidance of the honorific term. For a variety of reasons, doctors and nurses pursue different, conflicting moral agendas. The two professions are formed through different selection procedures; doctors are mostly men (though the plurality is rapidly shrinking), while nurses are mostly women; doctors are trained in a physiological model of disease; doctors have vastly more power; doctors do very different work; and, finally, doctors hold the legal responsibility for the patient's well-being, while nurses carry much of the day-to-day work of patient care. And nurses, unlike physicians, are often afraid of being "written up" (disciplined) or of losing their jobs or their licenses. Some conflicts erupt from an unwanted intrusion into the nurse's work: for instance, consider the complaint of a kidney dialysis nurse that a physician came into a patient's room during dialysis and began "fiddling with the catheter, which I had gotten just right," and messed it up. "Then he wanted me to come in right then and fix it, and I was doing other things. He had no business being in there." [Interview] It has often been said that physicians focus on cure, while nurses aim to care; it can be added that physicians are largely rewarded for scientific expertise, nurses for organizational skills. The different nature of their tasks can make common ground hard to find. For all these reasons, physicians and nurses are often at odds about what

should be done and why. The ideal of doctor and nurse working as a "team" is only an ideal. ("Empirical studies, however, show that nurses and physicians are not sharing colleagues; rather, they work side by side with severely limited communication and minimal interaction.")[9] Doctors often pursue goals that differ from those of nurses, and the resulting clash provokes arguments voiced in ethical terms:

—Physicians tend to be more aggressive than nurses in treating patients who are terminally ill. Although doctors vary in their willingness to continue invasive, costly treatment of terminal patients, they generally hesitate to let nurses treat terminal patients with only palliative care; nurses are more willing. This difference may result from the physician's sense of legal and personal responsibility for the case, the nurse's round-the-clock witnessing of the patient's suffering and the family's wishes, or the physician's strong orientation to the physiological outcomes rather than the personal experience of the patient. In any case, arguments over how much to treat hopeless cases are a staple of ethical conflict between nurses and doctors.

—The teaching function in hospitals often interferes with patient care, to the dismay of nurses. Physicians in training— that is, interns and residents in their first few years out of medical school—use the teaching hospital (the "learning hospital" might be more accurate) as a site for learn-by-doing medicine, in which relatively unpracticed physicians learn their craft by practicing on the bodies of patients, especially the indigent who, in effect, pay for treatment with their personal and bodily dignity:

> Intern is trying to start a triple-lumen catheter [a narrow tube with three different channels inside it], threading it into a femoral vein [in the thigh], up toward the heart. She tried first one leg, then the other, couldn't get the line in.
>
> Blood is all over the patient's legs, very hard to maintain the sterile field around the wounds. Intern, on her second day of work without rest, looks exhausted and dismayed; the nurses outside the room are rolling their eyes, say that "[the intern] thinks it's supposed to be like this," all the blood and such.

9. Benjamin and Curtis, *Ethics in Nursing,* p. 85.

Finally, the senior resident on the floor comes in and finishes the procedure. Was there a consent form signed for the procedure? No. "Well, we'll get it later," says the resident. [Field Notes]

A code (a resuscitation effort) may be called on a hopeless patient to provide the learning experience for the residents, who will need to know the procedure to save future lives. Especially valuable is the opportunity to learn to intubate—put an endotracheal tube down the throat to the lungs, for the ventilator.

—The prestige and lavish funding of high-tech science often drives medical action in ways that nurses resent. Researchers make their careers off the new, the rare, the extraordinary and dramatic medical cases. But most cases are not unusual or dramatic. Nurses take care of all the patients and are most absorbed in the routine activities of the hospitals. Medical researchers, on the other hand, focus on the unusual or especially difficult case and put their time, energy, and money into those cases. Nurses object to this imbalance:

I had a patient . . . he had radical neck surgery and he was so deformed you can't believe. He went through such a psychiatric episode from it that he's like a vegetable. So what good was it? . . .

It's a money-making business. [Patients] go [into the hospital] for treatment and they have a lot of money, and therefore they get treatment that maybe might not have been totally needed . . . Somebody's making a great deal of money off them. [Interview]

Andrew Jameton has nicely summarized the reality of prestige allocation among health professionals and its relation to science:

If health professionals were mainly concerned with public health and overall welfare, then they would develop and honor the skills most useful in maintaining these . . .

If health professionals were mainly concerned with doing the most obvious and immediate good for patients, they would emphasize skills in caring for and comforting the sick, that is, palliation of symptoms and relief of pain, since most diseases are still either incurable or self-limiting. If bedside care were in fact the most honored specialty, the prestige of the health professions would likely be the reverse of its present standing . . .

The most valued forms of competence currently tend to reflect scientific and technological interests—what people consider intellectually difficult, exciting, and challenging—rather than what is most directly related to patient good or to public health.[10]

—Finally, there is often a simple clash of the doctors' priorities versus those of the nurses. Physicians put a priority on diagnosis:

On the Neuro ICU, a pt in restraints, shaking back and forth every few seconds, severe head injury; gets very violent. The resident, Dr. R., won't sedate him or give him Pavulon (a paralytic which stops the seizures) because it makes assessment of the patient's condition impossible; they can't check his reactions, etc., if he's paralyzed. So when the patient goes down for a CT scan, the nurses are afraid he will become violent and hurt them (he is very violent).

If the patient is paralyzed to protect the nurses, then the docs can't assess him, and the resident will "get his ass chewed" by the attending. So instead, nurses get kicked and punched by this patient. Says one nurse, "Next time, we'll tell [Dr. R.], 'You transport him.'" [Field Notes]

Or the physicians, naturally enough, want their orders executed immediately, and nurses often have multiple "stat" orders to handle simultaneously, sometimes with conflicting goals between the medical specialties.

"The plastic guys want to make 'em look good," and so favor keeping burn patients in bed so the skin grafts will stick; "the general surgeons figure you just save 'em first, then go back and patch 'em up," and so it's best to have patients up and walking, to avoid pneumonia. It's an honest difference in style, but the result is arguments over treatment. [Interview]

10. Jameton, *Nursing Practice*, p. 85.

The priority of the doctor's "convenience" can sometimes be shown in remarkable insensitivity:

A man had cellulitis of the arm and the doctor came in, he was making rounds . . . He said, "I'm gonna operate on Mr. Martinez." When we got to the bed there was no Mr. Martinez. He said, "Where is he?"
The patient was in the bathroom, and the doctor knocked on the door and said, "Mr. Martinez?" Poor Mr. Martinez, who was probably on the commode, yelled, "Yeah?" and the doctor said, "We're gonna take you to surgery tomorrow, OK?" and left.
[Laugh] And Mr. Martinez was going "Doctor, doctor!" [Interview]

2. *Nurses versus administrators.* If doctors are visible opponents to nurses, with clear professional differences, administrators are even more pervasive in their influence and less localizable as opponents. Their goals—financial solvency of the institution, for example—may strike the nurses as morally suspect, and their priorities even less plausible than those of physicians. Administrators want to raise money, cut costs, attract prominent physicians and their patients, enhance the physical beauty of the hospital grounds, erect more buildings, and manage, as they see it, the overall well-being and stability of the hospital institution. All of this may strike the harried floor nurse as nearly irrelevant. Floor nursing and hospital administration see the world through very different lenses, and the resulting arguments are often framed in moral terms.

But "administration" is a broad term, covering everyone from the president of the hospital to a twenty-five-year-old head nurse on the pediatric floor. Some administrators are "blue coats," young men in middle management positions wearing navy blazers, personnel specialists, accountants, or cost control experts, who have little if any direct experience in patient care, either medical or nursing. Others are nurses who have worked their way up the hierarchy and now run the largest departments in the hospital—middle-aged women who identify as nurses, though away from the bedside for many years. There is, among practicing nurses, a generalized animosity toward "administration," but feelings toward particular administrators range from strong antipathy to passionate discipleship. Despite the occasional reverence nurses feel toward a supervisor in their own area, however, the typical attitude toward administration is one of generalized distrust. Complaints, as nurses express them, take various forms:

—Administrators don't understand life in the trenches and are contemptuous of their subordinates. This is typically framed as "lack of support, that would have to be the number one problem." The reference here is not to financial support but moral and organizational support. This may be the single major issue in nurses' dissatisfaction with their work—the feeling, expressed in many ways, that those around and above them don't appreciate what they do.

> Some assistant director [of nursing, an administrator] comes along, supposed to talk with you about your problems, and she's wearing this high-fashion outfit. You've been slopping around with bedpans. How is she supposed to understand my problems? [Interview]

Nurses complain that administrators "up there in their air-conditioned offices" (this said on a floor that was sweltering in the summertime) don't understand.

> "They give us ice cream cones once a year [at a social event], and we're supposed to feel better," says one. "I hate it"—the patronization, the inequity. "There's a caste system here, the aides and the unit secretaries are the untouchables; the staff nurses [are the next level up]. 'Well, maybe we'll say hello to them [think administrators].'" Administrators work a normal 8-hour day and leave behind the problems when they go home.
> "Ever try to get out of that parking lot at 5:00? It's jammed. They [administrators] all leave right at 5:00. You don't see *them* staying late." [Interview]

Sometimes administrators' pettiness is astonishing. In one meeting, a high administrator berated a group of head nurses about their "bulletin board management." Head nurses should, they were told, check out everything that is put on the bulletin boards on their floor, initialing each approved item and removing "the latest recipe for tuna salad," recruitment letters for other hospitals, chain letters, and other "inappropriate" items. This was the entire agenda of a weekly management meeting in an important [surgical] nursing area. Or, for another example, one head nurse I interviewed worked twenty-six hours straight, then slept four hours; then she worked eighteen hours more. A day later she received an official warning regarding her "failure to do paperwork on time." In yet another episode, overworked head nurses and supervisors were required to attend seminars and complete workbooks on "effective management"—but with no relief from the real difficulties of their jobs. In some cases, higher administrators deliberately cut themselves off from their people:

> Vice president's secretary, on phone: "Just a minute, I'll see if he's in." [She switches to another line.] "Dr. L——, M—— E—— is on the other line. Do you want to talk to her?"
> [And back to the first line] "I'm sorry, he was in earlier, but he's not around now." [Field Notes]

Here is the vice president of the hospital turning away a call from one of his own direct subordinates in nursing, with an outright lie. Poor management is not, of course, peculiar to hospitals; but here complaints about it seem to take on a distinctively moral tone.

—Administration, for whatever reasons, pours the most resources into the least productive areas. Hospitals spend lavishly on highly visible, glamorous services such as "Life Flight" helicopter rescue programs, MRI (Magnetic Resonance Imagery) scanning devices which cost millions of dollars each, organ transplant programs, and the like. But money for transplantation, for instance, is really money for medical research, to attract prestigious doctors; it is *not* an efficient way to preserve the health of the general population. Glamour services appeal to renowned physicians, generate publicity for the hospital, and may attract dollars from donors, but their direct impact on patient health in many cases is minimal.[11] High-tech medicine, such as is practiced in Intensive Care Units, soaks up huge amounts of money which could perhaps be more effi-

11. On the variable efficacy of clinical medicine generally, see Thomas Mc-Keown, *The Role of Medicine: Dream, Mirage or Nemesis?* (Princeton, NJ: Princeton University Press, 1979).

ciently used elsewhere. In Infant Care Units, nurses complain that "we don't have any money for prenatal care for these women, but we have enough money to keep her [hopelessly premature] fetus alive . . . They can't get their prenatal care or their transportation for prenatal care, and it would be so simple to prevent so many things . . . Yet we have millions of dollars to spend on a fetus . . . You're spending 3 million dollars and wrecking me emotionally, to send a kid home to people who are [eventually] gonna kill him" [Interview].

Then, too, money and people are expended on cosmetic upkeep of the hospital, in ways that sometimes actually interfere with daily work:

> In the Newborn Unit at H. Hospital, janitors come in at all hours with floor buffing machines—make a lot of noise so babies can't sleep. The nurses have complained and are told that patient satisfaction surveys show that *parents* (of the infants here) are very impressed with how nice [the floor tiles] of the unit look. When nurses complained that there was too much noise from the machines (you can't even hear people talk over it), and that they need another housekeeper since the garbage cans are often full and go unemptied, they are told that the floor buffing is more important! [Field Notes and Interview]

And this occurs while nurses who carry out the mundane, but necessary, day-to-day work on medical floors can't get basic supplies:

> All the penny-ante stuff—we can't get stickup notes, basic little things. It's penny-pinching, but you know, they'll tear up a whole big piece of land out there or redo the administration building so it's fancy for them. [Interview]

One nurse on a labor and delivery unit complains that administration provides the cheapest basic supplies—bandage tape that causes a skin rash, soap that causes skin sloughing (but sells for two cents a bottle)—while pouring hundreds of thousands of dollars into the latest medical technology. Another tells of repeated meetings and memos about the importance of infection control, but the sinks are filthy and the soap provided for nurses to scrub with causes a rash—so people don't use it, and infections spread. In all of these cases, an effort to save little bits of money can cause problems, while major expenditures produce relatively little in the way of true health care improvement.

—Administration imposes bureaucratic red tape which actively impedes the important work of nurses. The target of this complaint is made visible in the seventy-six multiplicate forms in plastic trays over the unit clerk's desk at Southwestern Medical Center; or in the eleven differently colored (pink, green, brown, orange, etc.) index cards taped over the clerk's desk, listing the members of the different "teams" of house staff who come trooping through the floor in the course of a day. It is evidenced by the twenty-two forms (no exaggeration) new employees at Southwestern must fill out—including one that verifies that the new employee has signed the previous form. Or the three weeks to get a telephone in one's office, or the keys to one's own office, or the six months to get a parking sticker, or the mandatory fingerprinting of new employees followed by a police inquiry ("We just want to make sure you haven't done anything wrong!" I was told). There are, finally, the computerized patient records, which allow anyone with the right code words to access any patient file (one nurse, herself a patient, asked her physician to omit personal information from her record, so everyone else in the hospital wouldn't know about it).

Some of these practices are inevitable, but some aren't. Many are legally mandated (consent forms, certain records, e.g.); many others allow the large hospital to function without constant interdepartment communication. Less excusable, though, are the "absolutely absurd" (as one nurse says) policies which through ignorance or insensitivity actually impede patient care, or, as exemplified in the following field notes and in Kraegel and Kachoyeanos, are simply cruel:

> The nurses repeatedly received a "valuables form" from the business office for a just-admitted patient: "The form needs to be signed," they were told. But the patient was paralyzed—and there was no provision for a patient who physically *couldn't* sign the form. [Field Notes]
>
> I remember helping a young nurse deal with her own bone cancer. She wanted to be a code—that is, to receive life-support measures if she stopped breathing. She was receiving morphine

for pain through a continuous intravenous drip. Our current nursing policy stated that a patient couldn't have a morphine drip unless she was a no-code. When the staff found out she was a code, they discontinued the drip. They attempted to talk her into a no-code so they could start the morphine drip again. It was like saying, "We'll take care of you and give you pain medication only if you'll agree to die."[12]

—Administration is to blame (some nurses feel) for the shortage of nurses in the hospital. A Neurosurgical ICU head nurse complains of 1–2 (nurse to patient) coverage on 1–1 patients. "One of them's gonna die because we aren't there," she says. Too much can happen when the nurse is out of the room; it's too easy to botch medication orders when you have lots of patients and no time to consider the various dosages and mixtures of pills and fluids being pushed.

Indeed, short staffing of nursing units is endemic to most American hospitals, and certainly to the ones studied for this book.

She's only had eight hours sick time in two years here. But in the past three Sundays, she was called in to work for lack of Ns . . .

This past Sunday (Easter) they called her in the middle of the day to come in: "I sat there and cried." [Interview]

P. [a head nurse in ICU] gets a call at 5:30 P.M.—new pt coming in. She doesn't have a nurse to cover it—if she can't find someone, she'll have to stay herself (making a 24-hour shift). [Field Notes]

I've been on 6–7 different floors here so far . . . in MICU staffing is a problem, but I've never actually seen them short a person. On all others, staffing and scheduling is a continuing problem. [Field Notes]

In 1979, in another hospital in another part of the country, the complaints were the same:

In arguments over unionization, the issue rarely seemed to be salaries, which many nurses say are good, and was almost always

12. Kraegel and Kachoyeanos, "*Just a Nurse*," p. 112, from an interview with a nurse.

working conditions, primarily staffing . . . one of the constant
complaints is that there aren't enough nurses to properly run
the patient care units.[13]

This shortage of nurses poses one of the great moral problems for nursing. Nurses feel that they don't have the time or
the people to care for all the sick patients who come into the
hospital. Many nurses feel a diffuse hostility to "administration" and blame it for a range of difficulties: the bureaucracy,
the mismanagement, the understaffing. Again, these conflicts
are not regarded as simple disagreements or priorities but often as real moral conflicts.

3. *Nurses versus the health care system.* Sometimes the nurse's
adversary is less defined than particular people, or even than
a class of "administrators" or "doctors." Sometimes—and
nurses put it this way—the enemy is "the system," the bureaucracy, the medical insurers, the government, the economic system of the United States, or the American health care system
(if it is a "system" at all and not simply chaos). Many ethical
problems faced by nurses are generated, as they see it, by the
macroscopic constraints under which they work. Organized
health care in America comprises a huge complex of competing interests and constituencies, each with its own imperatives,
and nurses often feel that their own problems result from the
actions of those other groups. Students sometimes reify this
"system," believing that it can act, and move, and interfere
with nurses doing their work. But of course "the system" is
really only an abstract way of referring to a complex of real
people and organizations carrying out multiple tasks, the results of which are often unintended, and which together can
give the appearance (since no one planned them) of a single
entity. Several of these forces can be clearly identified, and
their effects on nurses clearly stated:

—The complexity of the hospital organization can be the
nurse's adversary. This applies both inside and outside the
hospital proper. Inside, there are ICUs, Geriatric Units, laboratories, social work offices, billing departments, X-ray techni-

---

13. Daniel F. Chambliss, *The Bounds of Responsibility: A Study in the Social Psychology of Nursing Ethics* (Ph.D. diss., Yale University, 1982), p. 28.

cians, supply rooms, and a host of medical specialties to deal with any single patient admitted. The nurse must deal with all of these. The patient is approached and processed by many or all of these various parties. A patient may receive as many as 20–30 pills in a cup several times a day, and the nurse must ensure that the dosages and their timing are correct. On one floor I visited, nurses had a brief discussion one day trying to figure out whose urine was in a specimen bottle being sent to the lab (someone forgot to label it immediately). Dissimilar patients may be treated alike, as when Foley catheters (into the bladder) are used on all ICU patients so the nurses don't have to be constantly changing diapers—even though in half of all patients catheter use produces bladder infections. Efforts to manage the organizational complexity can thus create new problems.

Consider the generic case of a premature infant born of a poor teenage mother. Born perhaps twenty-five or twenty-six weeks into the pregnancy, such babies often have a very poor prognosis. They may be ventilator-dependent until their lungs stiffen, "turn to leather," and are useless; they are often physically and mentally deformed. But many doctors "can't stop treating"; the mother, perhaps a drug user, blames herself and becomes the child's protector, demanding more from the nurses and refusing to discuss any options; the father, perhaps not married to the mother, often leaves her after quarreling; the mother's parents try to take over; the state welfare system pours enormous amounts of money into saving such babies; and the infant itself, unable to speak but feeling the pain, can have no say in the matter whatsoever. Such cases are common. Too many interested parties means no clear right answer.

—Complexity and the ensuing confusion of responsibility mean that problem patients can easily be "dumped." "To dump" is hospital slang for getting rid of an undesirable patient, one who is medically untreatable and a drain on the staff's energy.[14] Two examples of how the term is used:

> In ICU rounds this morning, during the resident's discussion of a pt who was at the end of useful ICU treatment, Dr. R.

14. "Turfing" is the synonym used in Shem, *The House of God.*

[attending physician] made a loudspeaker with his hands to his mouth and chanted as the resident was talking, "Dump—Dump—Dump" at least a half dozen times. Meaning: get this pt out of here. [Field Notes]

Many of the nurses at NGH believe the hospital is what they call a "dumping ground" for the rest of the state, a place to send the hopeless patients. [Field Notes]

Pressures to dump a patient can lead quite directly to malpractice:

In rounds today, Dr. C., the resident, was complaining about strict isolation policy on MRSA (staph infection) patients. Others—nurses, mostly, suggested that yes, it's a bother having to isolate these patients, but if they culture positive, that's that.

Dr. C. said, "Well, if you ever have some time, I'll show you a foolproof method for making *sure* the culture isn't positive." The intern sitting next to him lifted her hand as if holding a swab and waved it back and forth, saying, "Culture the air." [Field Notes]

A med student today reported in Dr. G.'s seminar that he had a pt with a recurrent staph infection who kept getting sent back to the hospital from the nursing home. The attending told the student, "I don't care what you do, just make sure the culture comes back negative." This was so the pt would be sent to the nursing home . . .

Several other med students reported being faced with the same thing—attendings telling them to fake lab results. They used the expression "culture the air." [Field Notes]

In these cases residents and med students were being told, straight out, to commit malpractice in order to dump undesirable patients onto some other part of the system.

—Sometimes the law itself encourages nurses to do wrong. Fears of malpractice litigation may drive physicians and nurses to be less than honest with their patients about their own failings;[15] workplace legislation designed with bus drivers in mind (not to work over eight hours, for instance) is blindly applied

15. For a dramatic example, see David Hilfiker, *Healing the Wounds* (New York: Penguin Books, 1987).

to nurses—and is routinely circumvented; "right-to-life" laws, such as the so-called Baby Doe regulations (requiring that anyone witnessing any form of "euthanasia" report it to the authorities), require continued treatment of hopeless patients and force the confrontation of the law and morality.[16] Parental notification laws mean that an admitting clerk at Southwestern Hospital could not admit a thirteen-year-old girl with a possible ectopic pregnancy—an immediately life-threatening problem—without a "note from her mother," and the girl went home in pain [Interview]. And in one recent legal case, when two medical students admitted to cheating on an exam—in an ethics course, no less—the court judgment reinstated them in school and forbade any school officials from discussing the case or mentioning it in the students' future letters of reference.[17] The law itself can be an obstacle to morality.

—The limitation of financial resources often forces nurses to act in ways they find inappropriate. In most Western democracies, the health care system is funded by a single payer, with consequent administrative simplicity and equity of access to all patients. In America, we have an incredible variety of payers, from generous private insurance to underfunded Medicaid programs, with a resulting variety of access and quality of care. There is no equity in the system. We have private for-profit hospitals, luxurious in their accommodations, which market themselves to well-heeled, fully insured, and comparatively healthy (young, upper-class) patient populations. Such hospitals especially emphasize more profitable medical care such as heart bypass surgery and dialysis units. With the rise of these profit-making hospitals, public charity hospitals become increasingly burdened with nonpaying patients and are buried under higher and higher costs. In this trend, the nurse is caught between professional standards of competent care and the limited resources she is given to provide it.

Under such conditions, cost-cutting is a pervasive theme of the nurse's worklife. And costs are high: in 1990, an ICU bed in Southwestern Medical Center ran $700 a day for the

16. See Chapter 6 for details.
17. I was told of the details of the case by people who know the participants.

bed, $500 a day for the monitor that read off blood pressure and vital signs, and $550 a day for a ventilator. Most patients in the unit were using all of these. In another nearby unit, a large hand-lettered sign in the nurses' lounge reminds them of the cost of common laboratory tests:

DID YOU KNOW:
ABG [arterial blood gases] $36.00
c [with] [electro]Lytes   8.00
c Glucose   10.00
c O$_2$ SAT.   15.00
TOTAL (for everything) $69.00 [Field Notes]

And these pressures can lead to cutting corners:

> While prepping to put in a Swan [a Swan-Ganz catheter is fed through an artery to the heart to measure the pumping ability of the left ventricle], Dr. B. was asked by nurses if he wanted a surgical gown (in sterile package, wraparound); he said no, and put on a hair bonnet, scrubbed, then gloved, and tried to insert the catheter into the femoral artery. While prepping, he explained to me that while he should wear the gown, scrub gowns cost $50 apiece—"That's high-quality paper there," and "That's where your and my insurance money is going." [Field Notes]

Or in the Operating Room:

> Doctor, closing pt after a ventral hernia operation: "I need more staples."
> Nurse: "I'll get another staple gun."
> Doctor: "No, don't do that. Each one of these costs $35."
> The closing looks awful—rough, bulging—no plastic surgery job, that's for sure. Patient has previous gunshot wound, pancreatitis. [Field Notes]

So while costs are driven up by legal pressures—defensive medicine against malpractice suits, for instance—and by the complexity of the system, the redundancy of tests, and the profitability of certain procedures, other financial pressures hold costs down. Nursing and medicine are caught in the middle of this conflict. In such a setting, money is often a salient issue:

In a unit meeting for Pediatric Rehabilitation are physicians, nurses, occupational therapists, social workers, the whole crowd. Social worker presenting case of 10-year-old spina bifida boy, badly disabled, behavior and medical problems, poor bowel and bladder function, learning disabilities of all sorts. After detailing all these, social worker said, "On the positive side, Bobby has incredible insurance"—and got a big laugh. [Field Notes]

In a variety of ways, the financial structure of health care promotes bizarre, ethically challenging, choices:

A badly disabled little girl needs rehabilitation, but as she improves and is discharged, the government program will not pay for her care at home—so she stays in the hospital, costing far more than is needed. [Field Notes]

In one private, for-profit hospital, nurses work around the clock to save a 26-week premature infant who is hopeless—but fully insured—while the hospital will not admit a 32-week preemie born to an indigent mother. (One nurse working on the unit quit in disgust.) [Interview]

There is no lack of money in the medical system; the problem is not a shortage of funds or lack of resources per se. But when budget cuts are made, nurses often feel it in their daily work—in the shortage of surgical gloves, the declining quality of bandage tape, the lack of staff and time for patients. At the same time, very visible, expensive, dramatic interventions (such as heart transplants) are taking place in the same medical center.

—Not all ethical problems, however, entail conflict with a definable interest group. There is another source of problems that must be mentioned: the entire host of general social problems in American society. A brief review of these will have to suffice here:

The unwed-teenager pregnancy rate fills obstetrics wards with fourteen-year-old girls who smoke and play radios, to the distress of the older, married women having (more or less) planned families.

The *high crime rate* sends to the hospitals increasing numbers of victims, both innocent and otherwise, who pose for nurses the issue of caring for people wounded in shootouts, paralyzed while holding up a convenience store, beaten by fellow drug dealers, or injured in an auto wreck while fleeing the police. Is it right to transfuse liters of valuable blood into a dangerous criminal, thus withholding that blood from some more innocent patient?

Serious *drug abuse* is imported into the hospital as a medical problem and yet is self-imposed. Should we continue to treat alcoholics who continue to drink? Is crack addiction an issue appropriately addressed by one-at-a-time hospitalization? While the wealthy go to a Betty Ford clinic, paying to have their problems defined as medical, the poor head for a charity hospital—and reinforce the staff's view of the moral decay of the lower classes.

The *AIDS epidemic,* for years ignored by a government wishing to avoid controversy—and perhaps disdainful of the "guilty" victims of the disease—claims multiplying numbers of victims who are increasingly poor and minority. Single hospitals in major cities have had hundreds of AIDS deaths already, with the number soaring. Yet public policy to prevent the spread of the virus remains undeveloped.

Poverty in America generates disease—TB, malnutrition problems, dental problems, as well as a host of psychiatric difficulties such as depression and the like—and restricts access to health care. Inside the hospital, private (insured) patients do often receive better treatment, even in the most impersonal of settings: "Insofar as middle-class and wealthy patients are likelier to have private physicians and poor patients are likelier to depend on housestaff, the uneven distribution of advocacy over the patient population reintroduces class distinctions even into the 'classless' setting of intensive care."[18]

Finally, perhaps the greatest single moral concern for the health professions today is, simply, the *mass exclusion* of tens of millions of people from the system altogether.

CONCLUSION

The ethical problems of nursing, then, are neither random occurrences nor are they individual dilemmas of particular

18. Zussman, *Intensive Care,* p. 216.

nurses. They are, rather, structurally created and occur in bulk. They arise when the goals of two professions clash, or when occupational groups have different motives, or when "the system"—probably at some point definable as a field of interest groups—thwarts the efforts of certain people to do what they see as their jobs.

This emphasis on group conflict differs from the usual approach of medical and nursing ethics. In the traditional scheme, ethical problems arise as dilemmas faced by individual practitioners, who perceive a conflict among their own values. Certainly, this does happen; nurses do face true dilemmas in their work. But more often, I think, the clash of groups provokes what are labeled ethical problems: "I've never been so emotionally depleted that I felt I wanted to stop nursing cancer patients. *They* aren't the problem—the *system* is. The number one problem in being a clinical specialist is lack of appreciation by the nurses you work with, superiors and peers. The power plays of the physicians."[19]

Several historical developments have produced a recent increase of nursing ethics issues. Most important is the weakening of physicians' previously monolithic power. "Although the changes have altered almost every aspect of the relationship between doctor and patient—indeed, between medicine and society—the essence can be succinctly summarized: the discretion that the profession [of medicine] once enjoyed has been increasingly circumscribed, with an almost bewildering number of parties and procedures participating in medical decision making."[20] As physicians' previous hegemony over health care has weakened, other parties—third party insurers, attorneys, family members, patients, doctors, administrators—have come to take a role in decision making. Ethical conflicts then proliferate. With multiple physicians managing the same patient, with health care "teams" in charge of a patient's care, with a wide variety of workers in many professions managing patients each day, fights are inevitable. And they often become moral debates.

19. Nurse interviewed in Kraegel and Kachoyeanos, "*Just a Nurse*," p. 109.
20. David J. Rothman, *Strangers at the Bedside: A History of How Law and Bioethics Transformed Medical Decision Making* (New York: Basic Books, 1991), p. 1.

This chapter has presented a sociologized view of ethics: *ethical problems in the hospital reflect divergences of interest among groups.* Ethical issues, particularly those that arise in nursing, are not intellectual puzzles to be solved with the aid of clearly elaborated "principles," such as respect for autonomy, non-maleficence, beneficence, and justice.[21] They are not abstract issues, solvable by appeals to logic, through academic research, or merely with "enhanced communication," although that may help. Ethical issues are not a mere competition of ideas; they are a competition of *people*, who have their various goals and methods. They represent real problems in organizational action, constrained by legal, economic, social, and personal peculiarities. Education, sensitivity, and awareness may marginally affect political alignments, but ethical problems are not solvable by changing people's thought. The problems are not inside people's heads.

Thus, the problems of nursing are similar to the problems faced by other subordinate employees. Most workers are not the boss. Most do not have the power or the time to sit back and mull over big abstract issues, comparing all the possible options, debating various principles of action and the morality of various views. Most of us will never sit on "ethics committees" comprising a range of disciplines; most of us, I think, do not have the luxury of facing "dilemmas" in which we have the freedom to pick one course of action or the other. Powerful people—for instance, traditional solo practice physicians— have dilemmas; the rest of us have problems. Nurses, like most employees in large organizations, work for someone else, respond to multiple bosses, manage multiple demands on their time, enjoy a limited time to think about things, and suffer pressure to get on with the job. The legal, economic, and medical problems they face are immediate. And often they are ordered to do things they believe to be wrong. They are embedded in a network of real people, and their ethical problems arise as real issues within that network.

Many of these problems revolve around the treatment of patients, often the least powerful people on the scene. Patients are seen differently by different factions in the hospital, and

21. As explained in Beauchamp and Childress, *Principles of Biomedical Ethics.*

the staff sees them differently than they see themselves. If I am sick, then first is *I:* then I am *sick.* But to the staff, a patient is *by definition* a sick person and hence an object for the medical organization to work on, an item to be processed, to be viewed through the same scientific ontology in which doctors begin their training by working on cadavers—pieces of dead meat— rather than by, say, talking with live people with problems.[22] The staff's practiced view of patients will be the subject of the next chapter.

---

22. Some medical colleges have recently begun to modify their curricula to remedy this.

FIVE

The Patient
as Object

In the previous chapter, I argued that many ethics debates are ideological manifestations of self-interested factional conflicts; therefore, the increasingly self-conscious, articulated, independent position of nursing has given rise to the growth of "ethical problems" in nursing. Nurses clash with doctors, administrators, and others, and differences are expressed in moral terms, as questions of ethics. In this way, the structure of the hospital and of conflicts within it determine what are called "ethical problems."

Nurses' most persistent challenges, though, arise in their dealings with a relatively weak and apparently almost defenseless party: patients. In particular, disputes arise over what a patient is—one might say, over the patients' ontological status. For a medical institution, the patient is an object to be processed in institutionalized ways and to be treated as a biomechanical entity. Patients are institutionally objectified: detached from their own lives and life stories, physically taken from their home settings, behaviorally managed as a conglomerate of discrete parts to be treated by different specialists. But patients often resist this treatment in a number of ways, and nurses and doctors try to overcome the institutional habit. But the habit remains nonetheless. In these cases, moral problems result not from the contingent structure of the hospital but from the prevalent style of scientific medical treatment. Contemporary medicine, almost by its nature, treats patients as medical objects. Patients resist, and the resulting conflicts express themselves as "ethical problems."

THE GAP BETWEEN PATIENTS AND STAFF

Staff and patients often begin their relationship separated by a huge cultural gap. Certain people work in the health professions; certain other people are most in need of their services. Even apart from health conditions, the two groups are dramatically different. Especially in large hospitals, the staff is young while the patients are old. Head nurses twenty-seven years of age run floors filled with eighty-year-old patients; residents of thirty perform surgery on patients who could be their own grandparents. The staff is highly educated, holding college and graduate degrees; patients are often uneducated, even illiterate. Add to this the ethnic differences as well, with predominantly white doctors and nurses caring for a disproportionate number of minority patients, or Jewish doctors and Catholic nurses treating Protestant patients.[1] Sometimes the staff disapproves of cultural differences in style:

> An old Chicano man, patient, in hospital gown, sitting on bed, moving very slowly. Three small kids (3 years old or so), other kids in T-shirts, athletic socks, etc., running around room, into hall, etc. Their parents (patient's children?) sitting and watching. Nurse at station says: "It's good these Hispanics have a family. Don't wind up in here alone with no one to visit." But "I don't know if it's always good, they never let the patient rest." [Field Notes]

Patients and staff also differ in social class. Doctors are often wealthy, and nurses are fairly well off (and steadily employed). Patients, in contrast, are disproportionately poor and suffer misfortunes which compound each other. Malnutrition weakens the immune system. Without medical insurance, patients struggle to find a willing physician. The family car—if there is one—is often broken down and can't make the long drive to the clinic; there's no one to stay home and watch the baby. The poor are more often crime victims. When their diseases are left untreated, one ailment leads to another: diabetes to kidney failure, an infection to gangrene, despair to drugs to AIDS. Seeing poor people in hospitals, a middle-class observer

---

1. Zussman also deals with this issue in *Intensive Care*, p. 65–66.

is astonished by the huge array of problems they suffer and bring with them, like dirty clothes and barefoot children, to sit for 6 hours in an emergency room. Many patients are society's undesirables; in a Neurosurgery Unit, a third of all patients are young men who've been in motorcycle crashes, often more than once, many wearing tattoos. ("Tattoos are a risk factor for neuro problems," jokes one nurse.) Or prisoners in the state penal system, given free medical care by law, generating new resentments among staff. ("They come in here wanting nose jobs!" claims one nurse. "That's our money paying for that.") Or pregnant teenagers:

> Nurse in Newborn Unit explaining to others how this baby came in [premature]: apparently mother's delivery was provoked when she "fell off a chair, and went to the school nurse."
> "The school nurse?" the other nurses laughed.
> "Yeah, and she also has chlamydia." The group kept egging on the nurse telling the story and laughing. [Field Notes]

Most patients, then, are nothing like the staff. Given the cultural and economic gaps between staff and patients, it is perhaps not surprising that staff frequently make moral judgments on the behavior of patients. Nurses rage about irresponsible mothers, mothers who don't take care of themselves and so damage their babies ("babies" is the term mostly used here, not infants, kids, patients, but "babies"); mothers often abuse drugs, drink too much, and do things that obviously (to the nurses) will produce a damaged, tragic child who will suffer terribly as a result. Mothers of many of the sick newborns are young teenagers, twelve- and thirteen- and fourteen-year-olds. One such mother would come in to visit bringing her own Barbie doll. And the mother of Baby Watson was fourteen when the child was born, fifteen when it was disconnected from the ventilator and allowed to die.

A few patients are young, educated, white, and well-off, and thus somewhat like the staff. Most, though, are quite different. But all are, crucially, patients, and this by itself may prove the greatest difference of all. By definition, patients are different; here begins their creation as medical objects.

THE MEDICAL CONCEPT OF DISEASE

The gap between staff and patients is not merely demographic or cultural, and more is involved here than differences in income or language, in religion or age. The patient has a broken leg, or a damaged heart, or colon cancer; as Samuel Shem has written, "The patient is the one with the disease."[2] This fact, definitive of what hospitals manage, fundamentally divides the staff from the patients. For all their arguments with each other, nurses and doctors remain on the near side of illness, talking about a patient who is "over there" in the bed. Patients are sick people who have been "admitted" to the hospital and now find themselves defined as being on the receiving end of the hospital's work. Patients wear uniforms (gowns) and sleep in hospital beds; their lives are detailed on charts, their bodies are open for relevant inspections. They fill a role in the hospital organization. It is fundamentally the designation of "patient" that establishes the gap between patients and staff.

Staff have good motivations for believing that by definition "we" are healthy and "they" are sick. They must believe that "this can't happen to me," especially when they spend their days watching helpless people suffer. "When somebody comes through and they're twenty-six years old and they have some unknown disease and they die, that bothers me. It's hard not to relate something like that to yourself." They may have escaped depression by convincing themselves of their immunity to the disease. Some health workers even choose their fields for its distance from their personal concerns: men going into gynecology, young people into geriatrics, and nurses working with premature infants.

What is the conception of disease, and of patienthood, that is imposed on patients? Basically, the hospital projects a quasi-scientific vision of reality. This includes many elements of the scientific style: reliance on chemistry and biology, reliance on quantitative measures, and a belief in the primacy of a physiological view of reality. At the same time, it accepts the validity

2. Shem, *The House of God*. The phrase, given as one of the "Laws of the House of God," is used throughout the book.

of empirical "clinical judgment." Medicine has a somewhat de-personalized vision, in which, as Renée Anspach says, staff actions "both reflect and create a world view in which biological processes exist apart from persons, observations can be separated from those who make them, and the knowledge obtained from measurement instruments has a validity independent of the persons who use and interpret this diagnostic technology."[3]

From such a perspective, detachment is a reasonable way to deal with patients. When illness is defined biologically, it's professionally reasonable for a gastroenterologist to say that "a colonoscopy's not a bad procedure," just a matter of inserting a long flexible tube up the rectum and into the colon for a careful inspection. Colonoscopy is useful for removing polyps and detecting early colon cancer, which is very curable in the early stages. "Not bad." (One is reminded of "the old clinical saw that a minor operation is an operation being performed on someone else.")[4] And it's reasonable for a medical manual's lengthy description of a Swan-Ganz pulmonary artery catheterization to make no mention whatsoever of the patient's experience. And it's reasonable also for an attending physician to stand and talk for about two minutes with an elderly woman with COPD (Chronic Obstructive Pulmonary Disease, for instance, emphysema), her eyes wide with fear, in an Intensive Care Unit. He explains to her the deadliness of her illness, and asks, "If you stop breathing, what do you want us to do?"

"You do what you think is best."

He tries again. She knows that to be on a ventilator, with a tube in her throat, is not pleasant. She also knows that to refuse this means death.

She answers again, "You do what you think is best." For the physician visiting a hall full of desperately ill patients, it was a reasonable question. [Field Notes]

---

3. Renée Anspach, "Notes on the Sociology of Medical Discourse: The Language of Case Presentation," *Journal of Health and Social Behavior* 29, no. 4 (1988), p. 373.
4. Rothman, *Strangers at the Bedside*, p. 80.

From the medical viewpoint, it is reasonable to believe that these technical problems have technical solutions.[5] And perhaps it is unreasonable for patients to make a fuss over other issues. Sociologist Renee Fox notes, in her ethnography of an experimental medical unit, that

> the stress of some of the procedures [patients] underwent seemed to be as much connected with "feelings" of being helpless, passive, and constrained that such procedures aroused in them, as with the physical discomfort they entailed.[6]

Even Fox, a sensitive and perceptive observer, herself once a polio patient, has put "feelings" in quotation marks; the term itself remains medically suspect.

But for the patient, the technical definition of illness is all a giant mistake. "[P]atients do not experience illness as symptoms that can be mapped empirically onto a medically diagnosed syndrome (unless they are medically oversocialized or hypochondriacal) . . . curing of the disease does not automatically cure the illness (that is, the human response to the symptom)."[7] Patients may feel, "I don't belong here; why am I walking into a cancer clinic?" "To the layman, [the body] is a sacred thing," not to be handled and used lightly; it is, though, "a different sort of object" to the physician.[8]

So when patients' complaints are irrelevant to the medically defined problem they are, well, just irrelevant. One nurse tells of a patient, long unconscious, waking up and saying, "My feet hurt." The nurse laughed as she recounted this example of patients' concern with "little things." When patients complain of the room being cold, or a needle hurting, some staff will label them "whiners" (and I've seen a number of nurses in one hospital wearing buttons that say "whiners," with a circle and cross-line drawn on it). From the medical view, patients' complaints—gowns open in the back, too many blood samples drawn, crowds of doctors going in and out of the room at all

5. Jameton, *Nursing Practice*, p. 254.
6. Fox, *Experiment Perilous*, p. 121.
7. Benner and Wrubel, *The Primacy of Caring*, p. 8.
8. Hughes, *Men and Their Work*, p. 35.

hours—are often seen as trivial. Such complaints are *not* about disease but about how the hospital treats its patients. When treated well, when the "small" things are handled, patients can lavish praise on staff, doctors, and nurses. (Zussman, I think, in this respect accepts the medical view, saying nurses offer only "small" kindnesses. Patients, like children, have little control over their lives in the hospital, and what appear to those in the "healthy" world as small kindnesses are, to those benefiting from them, quite substantial indeed.)[9] What the doctor treats, that is, is not what the patient suffers.

THE PATIENT CREATED AS OBJECT

The patient's transformation into an object of medical scrutiny begins with his or her removal to the hospital, and not only in the physical sense. To be treated, the patient must accept the medical world's view of disease and treatment.[10] On leaving home and entering the hospital, the patient relinquishes the right to decide what bothers him or her. Professionals now diagnose "the problem" and decide what's wrong—or, indeed, that perhaps there's "really" nothing wrong at all.[11]

The patient is first separated from home, work, and even from biography. For most, illness is abnormal; it is a pathology, an unusual breakdown in an otherwise healthy daily routine. "I'm not usually like this," patients may feel. Families, too, suffer because their loved one has a normal life outside; they see the suffering against a background of a (relatively) healthy life. But the staff have only a hazy picture of this background. Nurses are not surprised that Mr. Jones has a Foley catheter in his penis, or that Ms. Jackson has a nasogastric tube in her nose, or that all patients are punctured with needles a half-dozen times a day. It's part of "being a patient." Once admitted to the hospital, the "patient" is dressed in a gown and laid in a bed with a chart outside on the door. All else is set aside. It's

9. Zussman, *Intensive Care,* chap. 5.

10. See Rothman, *Strangers at the Bedside,* for the history of how this state of affairs came about.

11. For an excellent description, see S. Kay Toombs, "Disability and the Self: A Matter of Embodiment," unpublished paper, October 1990.

normal from then on for "patients" to be examined by teams of physicians, injected, given enemas, catheterized, and discussed in rounds. The patient is a *case,* one among many:

> . . . this routine
> Misery has made us into cases, the one case
> The one doctor cures forever . . .
> . . . Our little flock
> Of blue-smocked sufferers, in naked equality,
> Longs for each nurse and doctor who goes by
> Well dressed, to make friends with, single out the *I*
> That used to be, but we are indistinguishable.[12]

One becomes an object of looking and talking. Examples are familiar: the written history, the chart detailing everything done to the patient, the physicians' and nurses' notes, and the endless physical exams (sometimes several times in a day). Then there are the more invasive lookings: endoscopies, bronchoscopies, colonoscopies, eye, ear, and nose exams; the blood tests, X-rays, CAT scans, MRIs, and the cardiac catheterizations. Hospital life for patients is an endless round of being looked at, listened to, touched and poked and prodded. Other observers have drawn attention to this. " 'In the unit,' one resident explained, 'it is a little bit of a science project . . . that's basically what people are reduced to. It's blood pressure, temperature, respirations, and their cardiogram' . . . the patient vanishes in intensive care—not, of course, as an object of treatment but, in any meaningful sense, as a participant."[13] Or as Relman, quoted earlier, has said, "Constant artificial light, ceaseless activity, frequent emergencies, and the ever-present threat of death create an atmosphere that can unnerve even the most phlegmatic of patients. Some are so sick that they are unaware of their surroundings or simply forget the experience, but for others the ICU is a nightmare remembered all too well."[14]

The patient forfeits other rights, for instance, that of pri-

12. Randall Jarrell, "The X-Ray Waiting Room in the Hospital," in *The Complete Poems* (New York: Farrar, Straus & Giroux, 1969), p. 297.
13. Zussman, *Intensive Care,* p. 32.
14. Relman, quoted in ibid., p. 21.

vacy, and by virtue of patienthood seems to become *less,* not more, morally protected from others. Some examples:

> From a chair in the ICU, I can look right into the rooms of 4 sick people—a violation of their privacy. The double doors are usually wide open, with nurses going in and out. When I'm sick, I want more privacy, not less—but they get less. [Field Notes]
>
> Nurse came up to T—— R——, a clinical nurse specialist, and started asking her about a mutual acquaintance who was HIV positive—in the middle of the hall, lots of people around. T—— was appalled, "Let's just tell everybody." [Interview]

Of course, patients can benefit from becoming a standardized object of medical attention. For instance, despite occasional charges to the contrary,[15] I saw little evidence anywhere in my research that social "undesirables"—criminals, drug abusers, unpleasant people—were individually given lesser treatment than the respectable.[16] I say "individually" because, as a class, the poor receive much less solicitous care than those with full insurance, and are sometimes totally rejected by some physicians and hospitals. At the same time, many nurses I spoke with and watched in nonprofit teaching hospitals were deeply committed to giving full care, the best technical care possible, to even the most indigent of their patients; the same held, I think, for criminals. The nurses sometimes resented such work, but at the same time they took great professional pride in doing it. Zussman makes the point well: "If contemporary medicine is less personal, it is also more tolerant. It is prepared to offer help not only to the solid citizen or the blameless victim but also to those of more often questioned character. It is prepared to treat the drug user, the drinker, the diabetic who fails to take her insulin, the man with kidney disease who misses his appointments for dialysis, with the same principled indifference that is, in other circumstances, a source of strident criticism."[17]

15. See David Sudnow, *Passing On: The Social Organization of Dying* (Englewood Cliffs, NJ: Prentice-Hall, 1967).

16. Crane agrees. See Crane, *The Sanctity of Social Life,* p. 96 and chap. 3.

17. Zussman, *Intensive Care,* p. 30.

Surgery provides a clear example of how patients are treated as objects. In the operating room the patient is ritualistically transformed from living person to medical object, making even the most grisly invasions routine. Typically, the patient is unconscious for the operation, save for an initial greeting by the anesthesiologist before he or she gives the patient the general anesthetic. ("What is your name?" "Grace." "OK, Grace, I'm Dr. Rodriguez. I'll be here the whole time. Now just breathe deeply.") And so the patient really is little more than a piece of living flesh. (When the patient is awake, on a spinal anesthetic, a sign will usually be on the door into the operating room, "Patient Awake," to warn staff who may come in to be on their best behavior.) Objectification is heightened by the initial preparation in which the area to be operated on is clearly separated from the rest of the patient's body. The patient's body is first covered by sheets save for the area to be cut open (say, the lower right abdomen for an appendectomy). That area is left bare; is shaved of hair; is cleansed thoroughly with a disinfectant solution; and is finally covered with a thin tight sheet of plastic, like you would use to cover leftover food. A drapery is put down between the patient's head (where the anesthesiologist sits) and the rest of the body, thus furthering the sense that "this is not a person." Even when a patient is awake, much can happen at the far end of the body—such as toes being amputated—while the patient chats away amiably with the anesthesiologist up at the head. Thus, there is little sense that the target tissue is fully human.

As I described in Chapter One, once the patient is anesthetized, the surgeons treat flesh as a careful chef might treat a piece of turkey being prepared for a Thanksgiving dinner. They slice, cut, sever; they pull on skin, muscles, sinews. They encounter fat, which looks just like it does in a turkey—yellow and greasy, it's the same stuff; they push fingers and hands deep into the viscera, dig around with fingers (say, to find different organs, all packed in there together); they sometimes pry and heave to move intestines, pressing and prodding with no evident hesitation. The "person," the patient, at this point certainly looks like no person you've ever seen or known, and it's hard to think of this body as a human being. "The body is meat," as Anne Sexton said.[18] Surgery is a violent procedure, and no wonder that when the anesthesia wears off the patient is sore. And surgery is profoundly intimate, though conducted with little evident sense of that. For the patient, the prospect of it can be terrifying:

> Big guy (6'4", well over 200 lbs.)—[state prison system inmate] strapped onto the operating table, cruciform [arms on boards straight out to sides, for IV lines], about to be intubated by wimpy little anesthesiology resident with glasses. Patient looks very scared, visibly trembling. Seems to me I'm watching the neighborhood bully's worse nightmare. [Field Notes]

In two other functions of the hospital, patients are quite explicitly objectified and used in pursuit of goals other than their own restored health. These goals are the teaching of young doctors and nurses, and medical research. The use of current patients for teaching is justified as helping future patients. "The doctors are here to learn," nurses often say in teaching hospitals. The phrase shifts attention from what is happening now to an indefinite future. The good of the immediate patient is not the goal, then, but is a constraint on other work which seeks to train doctors to help future patients. In the meanwhile, some patients are obviously used:

> I've seen a pt have a pneumothorax because an intern went to put in a subclavian, and would cause a spontaneous pneumothorax. They gave it to him again, and let him try again on the other side, and he caused *another* pneumothorax. Now this pt has bilateral chest tubes, because the intern was practicing . . . [Interview]

> [Pt was] an elderly man who had cancer and had some fluid in his lungs . . . I was called upon to assist at a procedure where they take a large metal device and literally stick it into the rib cage, into the lungs, and they put in tubes, chest tubes. Now that's not a pleasant experience under the best of circumstances. And here they had an inexperienced resident who needed the experience of doing it. [Interview]

18. See Sexton, *All My Pretty Ones*, p. 13.

Similar cases occur frequently, where interns try multiple times to start an arterial line (putting a needle into an artery to measure blood pressure) or carry out other difficult and, for the patient, painful procedures. Some procedures can be learned on the recently deceased—for instance, intubation, the insertion of an endotracheal tube into the throat for mechanical ventilation of the lungs. Perhaps a harsher example is provided by a nurse who reported that her worst ethical problems were in a medical ICU:

> A guy bleeding out of his eyes and ears, hopeless, and in the code they'd say, "Let's try 5 compressions and see what happens." Or "Look at what this drug does to the heart." They did codes for no reason, on patients who were going to die anyway. Just experimenting. [Interview]

The patient here is clearly being treated as an object for another's purpose.

In clinical research, too, patients are used. A nurse may find that after giving an experimental drug to five of the thirty patients chosen for a study, the drug is actually doing harm. But new patients keep coming in, and, says one such nurse, the nurses think, "My God, we're going to have to use that drug again . . . it won't help the patient, just test the drugs." But "you have to give the drug anyway, even if it isn't working well, because you're a research nurse." A historian concurs, and cites an ethicist: "The force that drove medicine down this path was the investigators' thirst for more information, a thirst so overwhelming that it could violate the sanctity of the person. 'I do not believe,' insisted Ramsey, 'that either the codes of medical ethics or the physicians who have undertaken to comment on them . . . will suffice to withstand the omnivorous appetite of scientific research . . . that has momentum and a life of its own.'"[19] True, patients are required by law to give their "informed consent" before participating in a research project. But do patients understand what they have signed in an "informed consent" form? The form says that the patient has been told the risks and benefits of the operation or research, yet it is the staff that chooses how much to tell and

19. Rothman, *Strangers at the Bedside*, p. 96.

how optimistically to tell it.[20] Patients are possibly intimidated, probably in desperate condition, and certainly dependent on nurses and doctors. They have good reason to avoid angering the staff. So they are easily pressured to sign.

Diana Crane, a widely experienced medical sociologist, looked at the issue of pressuring patients to stay in research studies, and concluded,

> The patient's freedom to bring the experiment to an end if he has reached the physical or mental state where continuation of the experiment seems unendurable to him is likely to be transgressed in practice. The physician is reluctant to terminate an experiment before it is finished since he thereby loses his total investment of time and money in the patient as a research subject.[21]

In her ethnography of a research unit, Renée Fox is considerably more positive in her view of how patient's wishes are respected.[22] But, in any case, there seems to be some clear treatment of the patient as an object in any research protocol.

LIMITATIONS ON OBJECTIFICATION

Still, we should not overstate the objectification of patients. Even in the highly technicized ICUs, staff know personal information about their patients and form judgments of them as human beings. One evening two ICU nurses, Maggie and Ken, sat and shared their thoughts on the difficulty in this setting of recognizing patients as persons:

> "We chemically restrain a lot of 'em," says Ken, "so they don't give us a hard time. Just conk 'em out."
> "It's good to have a photo of them outside the hospital," says Maggie, just to know they have other lives. [Field Notes]

---

20. See the excellent discussions in both Charles Bosk, *All God's Mistakes: Genetic Counseling in a Pediatric Hospital* (Chicago: University of Chicago Press, 1992); and Anspach, *Deciding Who Lives*.

21. Crane, *The Sanctity of Social Life*, p. 184.

22. Compare Fox, *Experiment Perilous*, with chap. 8 of Crane's *The Sanctity of Social Life*.

Efforts to remember patients as people take many forms. In the unit just mentioned, one nurse, known widely as being excellent both in technique (starting IVs, for instance) and in attitude, habitually attends to "little things." She makes symbolic statements of respect for her patients, giving them a bit of ice when they're thirsty, for instance, or protecting their fragile modesty. This nurse was a participant in the following scene:

> Guy in DTs, thrashing about, being sedated; they're holding him down; afterward they change the sheets, wipe his bottom after he craps all over, throw a piece of sheet over his genitals; it came off several times while they were fighting with him. Each time, someone would put it back, almost a symbolic effort, not as though everybody there hadn't seen, just a little statement that they were aware this guy is tied down and naked. [Field Notes]

Staff members can try to respect the person when the person is hardly there. In a Newborn Unit, where nurses care for premature infants—tiny creatures, some born as many as ten weeks early—many of the bassinets are decorated with little baby things:

> A yellow Winnie the Pooh, a little pink lamb with a white face . . . ; a plastic-painted balloon over another, with "Get Well Soon" on it; "I'm a Boy" card or "I'm a Girl" card over each bassinet, hospital provided, with name. Often the surnames have been changed, crossed out and revised—mother's or father's name, they aren't sure, etc., ambiguous family relations a common phenomenon here. The little baby toys, lots of them in some cribs, none in others. One now has a musical mobile of plastic rings and balls that plays "Brahms's Lullaby"; this baby, on a ventilator, is very active and stimulated. Others, tiny little overgrown fetuses almost, lie on vent[ilator] asleep, curled up, tiny, with a little stuffed animal in the corner. [Field Notes]

If the Newborn Unit nurses work to reaffirm the human being behind the medical object, in the kidney dialysis ward little such effort is necessary. The treatment itself forces nurses and patients to see each as persons. The technology of dialysis is routine, and the chronic patients may come to the same hospital for treatments three times a week for as long as twenty years. And at every dialysis treatment, careful procedure is crucial to prevent infection. So nurses work closely with patients to help them to learn the details of their own care. And the nurses celebrate when patients complete the course of training in home dialysis:

> Just had a graduation party for John (pt) in dialysis, with cake, etc., certificate—a "diploma." Very much *not* like a disease here, an achievement—"congratulations," etc., "part of the family" feeling by staff. "See you all next week!" he said as leaving. [Field Notes]

Nurses here talk of patients and their families quite directly as friends and colleagues; these patients are far less readily "objectified."

In many other ways a patient's "real life" may become evident. Sometimes a patient will dress in street clothes and walk about the floor, part of the civilian world again. Or a terminal patient will refuse the standard "heroic" treatment, and a nurse finds, as one put it, that

> it's harder to watch someone die when they are just *there*, breathing, talking, awake, instead of with lots of lines and tubes, intubated . . . they look like a real person from the street . . . it's like a regular person is dying. [Interview]

Finally, doctors and nurses who themselves become patients challenge the idea that patients are "different." They are often problem patients, knowing too well what tests are appropriate and what lies are told:

> One nurse was admitted to the hospital to have her wisdom teeth removed. The pre-op nurse came in her room and gave her an injection to prepare her for the surgery.
> "What did you give me?" asked the now-patient.
> "Oh, just a little something to make you sleepy."
> Then, the nurse standing there said, "Do I know you from somewhere?"
> "I'm the head nurse on 4-East."
> The nurse, embarrassed, told her the medication. [Interview]

So from a number of causes—a deliberate effort, close long-term contact, some kind of personal identification—staff do often see their patients in less objectified ways.

THE PATIENT RESISTS

The patient is typically treated as an object, but he or she tends to be a *resistant* object. Patients have their own ideas about what's wrong with them, what causes their problems, and how their problems should be treated, all of which frequently contradict the medical understandings of disease and treatment. Three kinds of patients resist being the grateful, cooperative objects of medical intervention the staff would like to treat. They are the incompetent; the openly noncompliant; and, finally, the self-destructive.

The Incompetent
Some patients are truly "non compos mentis," not in touch with reality:

> Mrs. B., old lady, confused, is in the hallway with all her luggage, waiting, she says, "for a bus." One of the nurses gently shows her back into her room: "You're here now!" [Field Notes]

The very young, too, are incompetent, not knowing what is happening and thus unable to give consent. In this case treatment can only be paternalistic, to the distress even of participants:

> [Today I witnessed] the needle injection of local anesthetic into a newborn (3 weeks) baby's skull, so they could remove a shunt. The two residents doing it discussed whether a local anesthetic would be sufficient; a general would be dangerous. One said, "I can do it if you can." This exchange was carried out a couple of times. A nurse (man) stroked the infant's hand, talked softly to it, and calmed it immediately as they were setting up, putting in the IVs—hard to do, the veins are so small.
>
> The resident injected the local anesthetic. Everyone around was affected by the immediate widening of the baby's eyes as the needle first went in, and then the screaming. The resident doing it, though, was absolutely concentrated on the task. At one point

the female resident mentioned her concern, saying something about the whole point of anesthetic is to lessen pain, not to increase it. The baby was put in pain, couldn't have known any reason for it, was helpless to resist. [Field Notes]

On some floors, many patients are "incompetent" in various ways: geriatric floors with Alzheimer's patients, a newborn unit, or pediatric floors with young children all face this issue. Often in Neurosurgery ICUs, all patients are restrained—tied down—because they are brain damaged and out of control. Even commonly used sedative drugs can lessen the patient's competence:

> Nurse, of pt: "He doesn't seem really oriented."
> Other nurse: "How can he be? He's getting Demerol q 2 hours! [every 2 hours]." [Field Notes]

If these patients recover, they will be grateful for the care that helped them; they may regard their own previous state as one of "incompetence." But if sick people aren't rational, this means that the staff can do whatever they want, and the patient is helpless to resist. A discussion I once overheard among some advanced medical students revealed a seductive, if treacherous, logic:

1. The medical students assumed that they—or at least, the medical profession—knew what was best for the patients.

2. They debated whether or not patients were competent, that is, *they* decided which patients would decide on their own treatment options.

3. They sometimes declared a patient "incompetent" by reason of depression—for example, a cancer patient who tries to refuse a bone marrow transplant (with poor chance of success); med student says a patient is depressed, so "not competent" to refuse treatment.

4. Thus they regarded patients' depression, "incompetence," etc., as independent of the staff's actions (e.g., forced or pressured treatment).

5. One student in particular believed that if patients didn't accept the treatment suggested by medical personnel, the patient was prima facie incompetent; so the treatment should be done anyway.

This last position, which is not rare in medical settings, does offer a certain closure to debate. Either the patient agrees with the medical view, and so is competent, and the staff proceeds accordingly; or the patient rejects rational, scientific medical reasoning, and so is incompetent—and the staff proceeds anyway.[23]

In practice, competence is often measured by very quick-and-dirty "tests": What is your name? Where are you? What day is this? Whether or not the patient is competent is decided by the staff, an interested party, and sometimes in ways that approach the bizarre:

> Dr. M—, the resident, goes into patient's room, 11:00 *at night,* shakes him and says cheerily, "Mr. Johnson, wake up! *It's morning!*"
>
> He wakes.
>
> "Do you know where you are?" [Field Notes]

From Mr. Johnson's point of view, some of the *staff* may seem incompetent. But the greater power of the medical and nursing staff allows them to decide whose competence is in question, how competence will be judged, and by whom.

The Noncompliant

Many patients fail to cooperate with, or even actively resist, their prescribed medical regimen. Staff call them "noncompliant." They include lung cancer victims who continue to smoke, dialysis patients who drink too much water, hypertensives who eat salted potato chips, and diabetics who don't take care of their feet. It includes the heart patient who escapes his bed to go for walks, the malnourished old man who pulls out his intravenous line, and all those patients who don't faithfully take their prescribed medications. Examples can be heartrending:

> Pt, 32-year-old male, diabetic. Told to stick himself 4 times/day [with an injection of insulin], watch diet, etc. "He doesn't care,"

---

23. Jameton sees and critizes these same arguments: "There is a tendency . . . for some professionals to use the concept of competence selectively to identify patients who *refuse* treatment as incompetent . . . If *competent* effectively means *agrees with me* and *incompetent* means *disagrees with me,* we approach full or *strong* paternalism." *Nursing Practice,* p. 26.

says nurse. Got a staph infection of the penis; "We told him his pecker would fall off, he'd go blind, couldn't see pretty women." But he still won't do anything. "We tried everything," told him he'd feel better if he did, get renal failure if he didn't. He doesn't care. [Field Notes]

Large numbers of patients do not comply with their prescribed treatment. "The majority of patients do not take medications as prescribed, and at least 25 percent do not take them at all."[24] Nurses I interviewed estimated that 50 percent of their patients were "noncompliant" in some way.

To a sociologist, this widespread resistance sends a signal. If a few patients were "noncompliant," we could attribute it to their lack of intelligence, self-destructiveness, or poor personal relations with the staff. But if 50 percent of patients are considered to be noncompliant, resisting their treatment, not following the advice given, and generally subverting the aims of the medical staff, something more is happening than sheer truculence. Perhaps the two groups—staff and patients—have totally different goals in mind. "If the patient is mistrustful of the nurse's urging, this does not necessarily mean that the patient is irrational."[25] Medical sociologist Irving K. Zola, himself a chronic patient, writes more strongly in an essay on noncompliance:

> [I]t is no longer safe to assume that patients regard the treatment they are asked to undertake as being entirely "for their own good" and "in their best interests . . ." To "take one's medicine" is in no sense the "natural thing" for patients to do. If anything, a safer working assumption is that most patients regard much of their medical treatment as unwanted, intrusive, disruptive, and the manner in which it is given presumptuous.[26]

From the patient's point of view, to repeat, the *staff* may be boldly noncompliant with the patient's own wishes. But "noncompliance" in the hospital means "noncompliance with medical authority." The very term defines medical reality as the dominant one; all the other views are deviations from it.

24. Ibid., p. 179.
25. Ibid., p. 211.
26. Irving Zola, *Socio-Medical Inquiries*, pp. 216–217.

Once again, staff expect the patient to "come into" the medical world, and, when patients resist, this is considered a "problem."[27]

Many nurses and physicians do understand the patient's feelings. Some physicians routinely make the point to their medical students:

> Dr. B—— was the new attending. At one point they discussed a patient, a young woman with asthma who had been intubated in the ER against her will—"she really resisted, was noncompliant," etc.; so reported the resident. Said she was still noncompliant. But Dr. B—— said, "Sometimes if people are noncompliant, they have a reason." [Field Notes]

Finally, some "noncompliant" patients are openly hostile. These cases are unusual, but quite unpleasant.

> We had a patient up here two days ago who gave us an incredibly rough time. I mean, the guy was a bastard, in plain English. Nasty as nasty could be. And he died, he arrested and he died.
> . . . People didn't want to admit that they were glad to see the guy go. [Interview]

The Self-Destructive
Finally, some patients, far from being cooperative, are actively self-destructive, not random victims of random diseases.[28] Even without "blaming the victim," an observer must see that many patients smoke too much, drink too much, and use too many recreational drugs. Some illnesses result from dangerous lifestyles, or habits (among others, e.g., motorcycle accidents, venereal disease, some heart disease or intestinal problems). And some patients just try to kill themselves:

> A huge [300 lb.] woman got mad at her boyfriend, sprayed herself with hairspray, then set herself aflame. [In Burn Unit], 90 percent covered with burns. [Field Notes]

Most common of the broadly "self-destructive" patients are smokers and alcoholics. They are part of the larger group of

27. See ibid., p. 218.
28. See also Zussman, *Intensive Care*, p. 40.

users of drugs, legal and illegal, who eventually find themselves in the hospital:

> V—— C——, 40-year-old man, with GI bleeds. Knife scar on belly, tattoo on arm, drinks 24 beers a day [told doc "maybe a dozen," wife says 30. Ns guess two dozen average]. Another guy in unit about 50, beard, big tattoos, heavy drinker. Also GI bleeds. Another guy cocaine/IV drugs, took an OD [overdose] of Inderal and Darvocet from his mom's medicine cabinet, 31 years old. [Field Notes]

The staff believe, reasonably, that such patients are unable to make good decisions, unwilling to accept treatment, and all too ready to destroy themselves; and these attitudes are seen as moral deficits. These patients are not just "failing to comply"; they are actively resisting the basic values of health and recovery; they are rejecting what Parsons called "the sick role."[29] They don't *want* to be healthy. To say the least, this is frustrating for the staff.

> Dr. M——, the resident, talks with other docs across the pt in bed (awake but intubated), as if pt not there. "We can do our best for him, but we can't save his life every time, if he's going to drink himself to death." [Field Notes]

Of course, the patient's symptoms here are less those of a disease and more those of a ruined life. But medicine can't treat that.

Which is exactly my point. *Medicine needs the object it can treat*—the defined problem, the curable disease, the grateful patient who believes in the doctor, the nurses, and the hospital. Patients who are not this sort of object (who instead are chronic, incurable, recalcitrant, or noncompliant) challenge more than medicine's effectiveness. They challenge its entire worldview.[30]

---

29. Talcott Parsons, *The Social System* (New York: Free Press, 1951), chap. 10.

30. Note: a final, strange case of the patient as a resistant object was revealed by a nurse in a neurosurgery unit, speaking of patients whose organs were to be "harvested" for transplants. One must wait until the patient is brain dead before taking the organs; and yet then, of course, the rest of the body has to be preserved. This is tricky. As the nurse said succinctly, "It's harder to keep 'em alive after they're dead." [Field Notes]

Again, we see a conflict between constituencies with different agendas. The issues of incompetence, noncompliance, and self-destructiveness all hinge on systematic differences of view between nurses and other staff members, on the one hand, and patients, on the other. This is not to recommend the patients' viewpoint. But in practice, it is medicine's power over patients, not the scientific legitimacy of its approach, that leads to its success in these arguments. The nurses and doctors are in charge here, so their view of what is right prevails.

CONTROLLING THE PATIENT

Because patients resist being treated like objects, the staff must work at controlling them. Control techniques range from gentle suggestions that "this will only hurt a little" to restraints put on violent patients who try to hurt themselves or other people (some psychiatric patients are suicidal; some neurology patients are hallucinatory and try to jump out of windows). Often nurses must negotiate between what patients want and what patients should get, making the sort of deals parents make with their children ("If you're good now, you can go for a walk later"). They persuade patients to stop smoking, to report symptoms promptly, to take their medications, to respect their prescribed dietary limits, to stay in the hospital until properly discharged, and not to pull out their IV lines. Nurses are responsible for maintaining such patient discipline. Doctors may talk angrily about patients' "noncompliance," but face-to-face it is a nurse who has to get Mrs. Jones to take her medication.

Some common elements of hospital care are designed to control difficult patients, protecting them from hurting themselves and others. Standard devices include "Posey belts," for preventing patients from falling out of bed, or leather restraints for patients who are badly disoriented or violent. Painkilling drugs are also part of the regimen; a patient's suffering can disrupt the work flow and thus needs controlling.[31] In ICUs, patients are also controlled with amnesiac drugs such as Versed. "You'll hear a lot of ICU nurses say—and this sounds

31. Barney Glaser and Anselm Strauss, *Awareness of Dying* (New York: Aldine Publishing Co., 1965), p. 208.

terrible—sometimes it's a real hassle to have a patient who can talk . . . you've got somebody who's really sick, and you've been doing all this stuff, and all of a sudden they wake up and say, 'My feet hurt,' or something . . . Sometimes you just want a patient who's on Versed and is not going to talk to you" [Interview].

Staff can also control patients by limiting patients' information about their medical condition. Northern General Hospital is a spinal cord injury center for the state, and many of the patients are young male victims of motorcycle and diving accidents. They are angry at being in the hospital; they are also often paralyzed. The doctor sometimes won't say, "You can never walk." But the nurse knows, and the patient asks. "They know when they're not being told."[32] One nurse tells of avoiding a patient, or spending her brief visits in the room talking nonstop, hoping to escape being asked the question she doesn't want to answer. When she finishes up with the patient, she says hurriedly, "If you need anything, just let me know," and runs out. But she says, "The patient knows something is wrong if you aren't talking with him."

Families' questions are especially hard to avoid. A wife can run to the physician, or a brother can complain to the hospital's board of trustees. Preston puts the dilemma well:

> Nurses generally do not know what the physician has told the relatives of a given patient. At times, physicians lie to or mislead relatives; at other times, relatives misinterpret physician's statements. This misinformation places nurses in a bind when visitors seek assurance.[33]

Sometimes family members will be waiting in the hall to visit a patient when, unknown to them, the patient dies. Nurses aren't officially allowed to notify families of a death, so a corpse

---

32. This puts special strain on nurses: "[T]he closed context instituted by the physician permits him to avoid the potentially distressing scene that may follow an announcement to his patient, but subjects nurses to strain, for they must spend the most time with the unaware patient, guarding constantly against disclosure." Ibid., p. 45.

33. Ronald Philip Preston, *The Dilemmas of Care: Social and Nursing Adaptions to the Deformed, the Disabled, and the Aged* (New York: Elsevier, 1979), p. 148.

may lie in the room as family members wait outside. Meanwhile, the nurse hopes a doctor will come by, recognize what's happened, and tell the family. All she can say is, "You'd better wait to talk with the doctor before you go in."

Sometimes patients are told only "what the doctors feel like they can handle"; the staff sometimes lies to the patients.[34] Because of specialization in medicine, such lies may involve several doctors and nurses.

> One patient, a boy 16 years old, came into Northern General with a brain tumor. Three different attending physicians were on the case—a neurosurgeon, a pediatrician, and a hematologist. The boy didn't know he had cancer until the hematologist, unaware that the boy didn't know, said something about chemotherapy. The boy and his family were devastated.[35] [Interview]

Substantial evidence supports the contention that deception of patients is far less common now than it was in the early 1960s.[36] Over the eleven years of my research, it seemed that outright lying to patients became less common and was certainly less accepted among hospital staffs. There remains, though, the slanting or selective presentation of information in such a way as to influence patient decisions.[37]

Perhaps controlling patients by these means (restraints, drugs, limiting information) is justified. Many patients are genuinely incompetent and in no position to decide on their own appropriate treatment. As one physician, director of an ICU, says,

> What do you do: a patient comes in, septic, seizing like a maniac, can barely breathe, incoherent—how can we ever get his "informed consent" to anything? [Field Notes]

34. See Sissela Bok, *Lying* (New York: Vintage, 1979), chap. 15.

35. For further details on this issue, see Glaser and Strauss, *Awareness of Dying*, p. 31.

36. "When the 1960s began, almost all physicians (90 percent in one study) reported that their 'usual policy' was not to tell patients about a finding of cancer. By the close of the 1970s, an equal percentage reported that they usually did tell patients such a diagnosis." Rothman, *Strangers at the Bedside*, p. 147.

37. Bosk, *All God's Mistakes*, contains excellent examples.

Even when patients are coherent, control efforts may be used for the patient's own protection. One geriatric nurse explained that many attending physicians don't like using restraints on their elderly patients, but

> they aren't here to see what we deal with. Patients get out of bed, fall and break hips, ribs—then the family sues! Or the family complains about the restraints when patient is tied to prevent his/her pulling out lines, catheters, to stay in bed—so restraints come off, patient gets hurt, or leaves, walks out, gets hit by a car on the street—and the family sues! You can't win. [Field Notes]

In these cases, it's easy to see the staff's point of view. In others, it's more debatable.

The terror of being forcibly treated—of being reduced to a mere object of medical scrutiny and manipulation—filled nurses' own sleeping dreams:

> B—— H—— reports "nightmares about winding up in this unit: tied down, all these nurses doing stuff to me, being intubated." Also nightmares about her sister being here. "I'm bagging her [using an ambu-bag to sustain breathing] in a code, and I blow out her lung." [Field Notes]

> Y—— J—— said her recurring "bad dream" or nightmare was waking up in the Neurosurgery Unit, paralyzed, an ET [endotracheal] tube in her throat, an NG tube in her nose, defibrillation burns on her chest, and Dr. B—— [a particularly unpopular female neurosurgeon] standing over her saying brightly, "Show me 2 fingers! [a test of the patient's orientation and motor control]."

> She says, "I wake up screaming." [Field Notes]

PATIENTS' RIGHTS

At this point, the skeptical or dismayed reader may ask, "But don't patients have rights? And aren't these recognized by hospitals?"

Yes, in recent years many hospitals have adopted (and posted prominently) a "Patient's Bill of Rights." But one should recognize that such rights are *granted* to patients, not taken by them. Even here the organization maintains an upper hand. Indeed, the very idea of a "Patient's Bill of Rights" is peculiarly revealing of the system's inherent paternalism:[38]

—First, a Bill of Rights given by the hospital can be revoked by the hospital; it is presented as a gesture of good will, not a statement of legally enforced rights. If anything, such gestures put the weaker party that much more in the debt of the powerful.

—Second, like a consent decree in law, the Patient's Bill of Rights has about it the faint odor of guilt. It seems to say: "We will never do these things which we didn't really do in the first place," such as operating on unconsenting patients.

—Third, this beneficent giving of rights to the patient may only heighten the patient's sense of powerlessness, a reminder of what *could* happen.

It is interesting that in cases where patients have won the legal power to accept or reject medical judgment, they often go ahead and accept it. To some M.D.s I spoke with, this shows patients' "irrationality"; but perhaps, instead, it reveals that the patients' argument is not over the value of scientific medicine but over the control of it.

So even what appear as efforts for "patient's rights" can subtly reinforce the status of medicine. Consider the case of Dr. Jack Kevorkian, who in 1990 invented a device for helping willing patients commit suicide. A lively public debate ensued around whether this was appropriate medical (or even human) behavior. I would note here that Kevorkian's device, a metal frame with a series of IV bottles controlled by the "patient" pushing a button, is visibly a medical/technological machine. As a suicide method, it is obviously unlike the traditional revolver or carbon monoxide in a closed garage. The machine is designed, and prepared for the patient, by a licensed M.D.— Dr. Kevorkian, in the famous case. Presented as enhancing patient's control over when to die, Kevorkian's device, I suggest, in fact reinforces the medicalized vision and control of

38. See Rothman, *Strangers at the Bedside*, p. 146; and Jameton, *Intensive Care*, pp. 202–203.

death. Even suicide, it says, can be medically managed. You
just need the right doctor.[39]

The hospital, then, has its own priorities and habits, some
of which may directly conflict with those of the patient. Patients
entering a hospital—with thousands of employees, with a long
and distinguished tradition of medical science, a training center for the nation's finest young physicians—have little hope
that their opinions will count for much. They can expect to be
treated as objects—valuable ones, certainly—for processing,
something like a car on an assembly line. One person admits
them, another decides what they will eat, still another serves
their meals, another tries to cure their sicknesses, and another,
perhaps, comforts them in their grief. The extensive division
of labor subjects patients to "process production" in which each
member of the staff has some particular job to do on them.
This is entirely apart from the motivations or personal beliefs
of any particular doctor or nurse.

Reform efforts, as expressed in a Patient's Bill of Rights,
fail to address the fundamental issue: the powerful staff can
impose its view that the patient is a kind of object. And if
the patient is sick enough to wind up in Intensive Care, the
levels of abstraction from commonsense perception of problems grow. The patient may say, "I can't walk without becoming exhausted," but the "real" problem—as diagnosed by experts—becomes abnormal blood gas values, or pH levels, or
inadequate blood volumes in an artery from the heart. This
physiological reality becomes the medically recognized problem, and the patient's "personal" difficulties become "precipi-
tating factors." Medical doctors, by training, believe in physical
reality at the biological level; that's where disease for them
really exists, and that is where it can be treated.

CONCLUSION

Sometimes it seems that the hospital as an organization wants
to know everything it can about this physical object, the patient.
Perhaps this results from "defensive medicine," in which doc-

39. Lisa Belkin, "Doctor Tells of First Death Using Suicide Device," *New York
Times,* June 6, 1990.

tors try to prevent any malpractice suits by covering every possible contingency. Perhaps it results in part from a technological imperative, in which expensive machinery must be
frequently used to justify its purchase. The sources of this effort at "total knowledge" are multiple, and the effort itself is
evident in the endless quest for information on patients: tests,
exams, X-rays, MRIs, CAT scans, and catheterizations; in the
monitors hooked up, temperatures taken, blood pressures,
urine and stool output measured, food and water intake recorded; in the yearly checkup, the monthly breast self-exam,
the hearing and vision tests, dentists checking over and under
tongues for signs of cancer, blood tests, cholesterol tests, the
routine chest X-ray, the six-month dental X-rays, not to mention routine notings of height and weight. All of this searching
is conducted through an endless and seemingly increasing
array of "lookings-in"—in search of some diagnosis, perhaps,
or in the hope of finding something. The computerization of
records has only expedited the effort. The goal of all this looking seems to be an idealized "total viewing" of the patient, in
which everything is seen, recorded, and classified.

In psychiatry, a pioneer in this area, total observation
means that the patient's every action, every thought, and every
passing fantasy, is grist for the analyst's mill. In psychiatric
hospital wards it means that staff not only watch patients constantly, scrutinizing their every move (no wonder people in
such units are paranoid!), but also spend hours or days sitting
and talking about them.[40] One acute psychiatric floor, for instance, houses adolescents with serious problems such as depression, chronic drug abuse, or suicidal tendencies. The
nurses begin their day by making the rounds of patient rooms,
greeting each resident. A nurse charts how long each patient
slept ("6 1/2//8," i.e., 6-1/2 hours at night, 8 hours total in 24).
Nurses make rounds of rooms every thirty minutes or so to
"catch 'em sleeping," a practice that is discouraged. At the shift
change meeting, in a room crowded with nurses, aides, orderlies, interns, residents, and medical students, reports are given
on how much each patient ate at meals (80 percent, 10 percent,
etc.), how they have excreted ("Jimmy had two stools, one

40. Erving Goffman, *Asylums: Essays on the Social Situation of Mental Patients and
Other Inmates* (New York: Doubleday, 1961).

soft"), and how they are behaving (who is showing some "oppositional behavior" today). The entire staff can sit in on these meetings, in which any residual sense of the patient's privacy in the most personal matters disappears entirely.

In one sense, such scrutiny of patients can actually produce, or at least discover, illness that wasn't there previously. If you look closely enough, everyone has something medically "wrong" (one soft stool?), out of line, or away from the norm. When doctors begin to measure cholesterol, some people are found to have "high" cholesterol. If nurses record patients' sleeping hours, some will be found to sleep "too much." If neurosurgery patients stay in doorless rooms, one may discover that, as one nurse notes, "They masturbate all the time." (The nurse says, "What are you doing in there?" "Oh, nothing.") Behaviors common but hidden among nonpatients become items of note. And if, after all this looking, no immediate problem is found, one can be projected into the future—a mole could do this, a lump might become that—and so is born a new category of medical deviance: "at risk." The patient does not have a problem but might someday, and so needs treatment today—or at least more observation.

Patients' very first encounters with physicians typically begin with a nurse saying, "The doctor will see you now." That phrase, we now realize, is more true than we knew.[41] The ailing person, in becoming a patient, enters a world in which seeing, in the broad and deep senses, is the key to understanding; and in which perhaps even the rounds of examinations, tests, and recordings serve to keep the patient in his or her place, as an object of medical scrutiny.[42] Medical observation then becomes a ritual of power in which roles are recurrently played out, in a way reminiscent of how Michel Foucault describes the modern prison (or any disciplinary institution): "an interrogation without end, an investigation that would be extended without limit to a meticulous and even more analytical observation . . . a file that was never closed . . . the ruthless curiosity of an examina-

41. The idea was suggested to me by Dan Ryan, Jr.

42. The classic work on medical observation is Stanley Reiser, *Medicine and the Reign of Technology* (Cambridge: Cambridge University Press, 1978).

tion."[43] Here, the ritual of examination produces an object, or at least an object-as-treated: the patient. The patient becomes, as we have seen, a person *defined* as sick, regarded as open for inspection as needed, and treated with procedures appropriate for a delicate living organism but not for a sacred creature.

Nurses are active players in this process. They are physically close to patients; they see and hear and feel them. Nurses claim this contact as one of their own great values: they are the "eyes and ears" of the physician at the bedside. They are continually evaluating the patient, assessing her condition, watching and always recording what happens. The objectification of patients is not so much the personal decision of cunning nurses and physicians, nor certainly the official policy of oppressive hospitals. It's far more pervasive than that. I might even suggest, in concluding this chapter, that seeing and the objectification it entails are almost the heart of the medical system. This regarding of the patient as a certain kind of object—a resisting object, to be controlled—may itself be a defining characteristic of medicine's ontology. The dominant power of the staff makes objectification possible, and the patient's continuing resistance produces ethical problems for the staff, as they worry over how ethically to handle incompetent, noncompliant, or self-destructive patients.

In the previous chapter, I suggested that ethical issues are often the ideological manifestation of interest conflicts between different constituencies. In this chapter we have seen a conflict of a particular kind, in which the hospital staff, with the power to do so, wants to treat patients as one sort of creature; patients sometimes insist on being treated differently. Around arguments over the nature of patients and their problems grow the ethical issues of compliance, competence, and control. As we will see, nowhere are conflicts over the nature of the patient, and how he or she will be treated, greater than in the decision of how to deal with the dying human being.

---

43. Michel Foucault, *Discipline and Punish: The Birth of the Prison* (New York: Vintage Books, 1979), p. 227.

SIX

Death as
an Organizational Act

Even in the handling of death, the hospital routine continues. Patients die, and some nurses find death too troubling to handle. But the organization continues on its way. Work is still done, patients are still patients, procedures are still followed, and the system itself continues, despite the coming and going of patients and nurses. Neither the dying patient nor the troubled nurse disturbs the pattern. Hospital talk supports the reality that "everything's normal." In dealing with dying patients, say Glaser and Strauss, "It is customary [among staff and terminal patients] to talk about the daily routines . . . When something happens, or is said, that tends to expose the fiction that both parties are attempting to sustain [that the pt is not dying], then each must pretend that nothing has gone awry."[1]

In this chapter we will examine how hospitals manage the dying patient, and we will find that responsibility for handling of dying patients is often diffused across a variety of people.

> In MICU rounds, we got to Mr. Smith, who is not brain dead but is pretty seriously gone. He's 77, almost nonresponsive, but had a cough reflex yesterday. He's a No Code—no antibiotics, no lab tests, no CPR, no vasopressors. (The original order on chart read, "Pt is a No Code: No CPR, No Pressor, No Antiarhythmics, No Cardioversion.")
>
> The Fellow [in charge] just stopped the report on Smith early and said, "This is an ethics problem," and motioned to the intern to proceed to the next patient. "Ethics problem" here

1. Glaser and Strauss, *Awareness of Dying*, p. 73.

meant "not a medical problem, not for us to discuss, out of our hands," something like that. The Fellow was clearly not saying that this was of "deep moral concern" or anything like that. [Field Notes]

Responsibility here is displaced from individuals onto the formally organized collectivity. Suggested in such remarks is the presence of a new level of moral actor—the organization itself.

We shouldn't be surprised that the organization itself seems to act. Previous topics in this book—routinization, the acceptance of roles, and shaping the patient into an object— are all facets of "organizing" the hospital. In such an organization, ethical problems are not the dilemmas of an individual conscience but instead of the organization itself. As this new organizational actor is created,[2] morality is displaced from the level of individual choice to the level of intraorganizational conflict and choice. With the growth of organizational actors, we see the decline of individual morality, not so much because people "don't care" but because it doesn't matter if they do. Ethical decision making, as I suggested earlier, is in some ways a privilege reserved for the powerful. In a world dominated by large organizations, that means ethics is reserved for organizations. But can responsibility really be displaced onto the organization? Individual people retain their feelings; they face deeply troubling problems that aren't dismissed by saying "I'm just doing my job." For several reasons, displacement is especially difficult when nurses treat dying patients. Death is irreversible. There is no "treatment" for death the way there are for other conditions patients present. In addition, death is universal. Unlike any other condition staff will manage, death happens to everyone, and so nurses find it especially difficult to separate the patient out as an Other, as "unlike me." Certainly, the staff often believes that "this could never happen to me," but, of course, dying will indeed happen to all of them. Nurses sometimes say that to deal with dying patients one must confront the fact of one's own

---

2. See James S. Coleman, *Power and the Structure of Society* (New York: W. W. Norton, 1974), for a history of the concept of the organization as actor.

death. So in facing death the nurse cannot easily hide in her role of "nurse"; official patterns may seem inadequate as a guide to behavior. The dying patient destroys the promise of medical intervention and challenges the medical model of cure.

Still, death—or, certainly, "dying"—is ambiguous and can itself be managed in the organizational context. "That a person is 'dying' is not an altogether straightforward notion, given the possibility that in a manner of speaking it can properly be said of all persons that, from the moment of birth onward, they move closer to death each day."[3] Even at the biological level, "dead" is not an all-or-nothing concept. Different body parts—a foot, a kidney, even a lung—can die while the person remains alive. People can survive the permanent removal (and replacement) of their own heart. In hospitals, one can see a living body directly connected to what is patently a dead leg—a bizarre sight, to be sure, but not so rare.

The dying patient often is treated as any other; the patient's status as object is maintained even when treatment is "futile." (Recall the earlier example of the hopelessly ill man; the attending physician said, "If he codes, code him!") In the hospital, death is not allowed to interrupt the normal routine. The dying patient may be stepped around, avoided, or pointedly treated normally, as in this case with a newborn infant: "How I coped with it was I didn't think about too much. I just looked at the tasks at hand. You felt very task oriented, take your vital signs, change your tubes, suction your baby . . . give meds . . ." [Interview]. But for the most part, normality is maintained. "There was a lady that for all intents and purposes was dead! . . . Because her family . . . wanted everything done, that's what we did. So for essentially two weeks, we took care of a corpse" [Interview]. Even when dead the patient remained in the system.

A patient's dying can be handled in a variety of ways. The cases described here are of terribly ill patients, in whom death appears to be imminent. Patients in such conditions are often suffering terribly and often want staff to stop treating them.

3. Sudnow, *Passing On,* p. 61.

" 'Request' is too mild a term to describe this behavior: many patients actually beg and plead to be allowed to die."[4]

> . . . 65-year-old man with gastric cancer. This guy was a mess. He needed gastric lavage every hour, with iced saline, followed by Maalox. The man was hemorrhaging, internally bleeding . . . Whenever I went into the room to give some treatment, as soon as the iced saline went into his stomach, he would groan and grimace in agony and plead for me to stop. [Interview]

> I'll never forget this particular gentleman . . . He came into the hospital with a potassium level of 7.5, which is hyperkalemia, and that's very dangerous . . . So he needed what we call [kayexalating] enemas; it's the treatment of choice for hyperkalemia. Now this man was in terrible pain, and I'm very soft and I'm very sensitive and I don't like to see people suffer. And said something, you know, "Matthew, I need to give you kalexing [sic] enemas, ten, one after another [to draw out the excess potassium] . . ." The procedure in itself is exhausting . . . and I remember . . . he would say to me, "Cindy, please, kill me. Please stop this torture." [Interview]

> We had a young girl up here last year when I first started working here. She was twenty-six and had ovarian cancer. It was so terrible; they just kept doing more things to her. I mean she was full of cancer . . . One time they started to do a really big resuscitation on her, she had no blood pressure left, and they started giving her all these medications; the only people that were in there were the interns and residents because we all walked out on them. We couldn't do it anymore. She didn't even look human, she didn't resemble any type of a human being when she died, she was just so distorted and gross. [Interview]

Death may be bad but sometimes so is the treatment that delays it. One nurse, describing her first experience of caring for a hopelessly ill old man, said, "I came out of that experience believing there were things worse than death, and I was being asked to do them." Often the patients are not even conscious; they are alive only in some technical sense. "We've got drugs

4. Glaser and Strauss, *Awareness of Dying*, p. 217.

to make their blood pressure stay up and we've got drugs to keep their heart going, and we've got a ventilator to breathe for them . . . There's really no way of knowing whether these people are even in there . . . whether or not we're dealing with a corpse that we're giving an artificial blood pressure to" [Interview]. Aggressive treatments—use of vasopressors to keep blood pressure up, use of ventilators to take over breathing for the patients, manual compression of the heart—may in a clinical definition keep a patient alive, but,

> I mean, they can ventilate you, and they can keep you alive a long time, but you're still dead, right? [Interview]

Treatments for these patients range from the aggressive efforts to save, exemplified by cardiopulmonary resuscitation, down to a minimum of supportive care, medications, and even—though in exceedingly rare cases—the use of something like "active" euthanasia, which to my knowledge is never openly acknowledged in American hospitals. The remainder of this chapter will describe these options in sequence. In many cases, we will see how the responsibility for treatment is diffused among the staff, thus reinforcing an image of "the staff" or even "the hospital" as the effective moral actor.

THE RANGE OF TREATMENTS

Full Code
Several times a day, an announcement comes over the public address system at Northern General: "Code 5," the voice says, and adds the name of a unit or floor: "Code 5, 2-West." This means that on that unit a patient has arrested, breathing has stopped, a heart has failed. Heart *failure* is not usually a heart *stoppage*. What usually happens in some 85 percent of cases is that the heart goes into ventricular fibrillation ("V-fib"). This is like an athlete's muscle, totally exhausted: it doesn't collapse but begins to shiver, vibrate almost, in a soft but very rapid motion. Resuscitation procedures are designed to stop this quivering and get the heart back into a strong, steady beat. When a "code" is called (usually after a nurse has discovered the arrested patient), a team of doctors and nurses from around the hospital converge on the floor. A "code cart" full

of medicines and metal and rubber devices is wheeled into the patient's room. Doctors, nurses, aides, and curious medical students jam the room (in the daytime, says one nurse, "half the hospital shows up"). A red "arrest board" is slipped under the patient to give firm support, and the team goes to work on the body.[5]

One person, usually a respiratory therapist, inserts a hose into the mouth, down the trachea, and into the lungs, attaches a rubber "ambu-bag" to the outside end, and starts squeezing it to force air into the lungs. A physician cuts open the subclavian vein at the base of the neck and attaches an IV tube to it. The vein leads directly to the heart, and through it a variety of drugs are injected: sometimes sodium bicarbonate, to offset the blood acid produced by lack of oxygen; lidocaine, to lower the heart's receptiveness to the brain's electrical impulses so the muscles will contract less often but more strongly; and epinephrine (adrenaline) to increase the heart's contractive strength. One person, meanwhile, is pumping down rhythmically on the breastbone, trying to reset the heart into its natural contractions. If the pumping doesn't work, defibrillation ("buzzing") is tried: two greased electrode paddles are placed on the patient, one on the breastbone and the other under the arm or on the back. A strong current of electricity (400 watt-seconds, usually) is fired through the body, in hopes of clearing the electrical confusion in the heart muscles, so normal contractions can resume. The code activity usually lasts fifteen to thirty minutes but can continue for hours.

For the patient being worked on, a code is, as one nurse says, "not very nice." The physical punishment is tremendous.

> Hopefully, the patient passes out before the code so they don't know what's going on . . . They had a case once where a guy . . . was in V-tak [ventricular tachycardia] so they couldn't put him out, so he was awake while they were shocking him, and his chest looked like burned leather. They would watch him go under and say, "I'm sorry I have to do this," and they would punch him in the chest. [Interview]

5. The following description of CPR comes from my own observation of a number of codes as well as from written sources.

Occasionally someone will protest, but typically the doctors favor aggressive treatment, and they are in charge.[6] In practice, an average of around 15 percent of patients who are successfully resuscitated survive to leave the hospital.[7] Most successful CPRs, it seems, are performed on otherwise healthy patients who have suffered a first heart attack. But codes are usually carried through with no thought of stopping. Reasonably enough, the issue never comes up.

But even in hopeless cases, a number of habits and rationales drive the full code:

1. "If you sit and think about what to do during a code, you never get things done . . . You're most mechanical when there's the most to do." Codes are desperate and exciting. The technical problems alone are enough to keep a good nurse fully occupied without ever worrying over philosophical questions of the value of life. The nurse may find herself, as one puts it, "getting into the techniques of it, giving the shots, the machines, calling the docs . . . " There's no time for making decisions.

2. To many people, life itself is an absolute value. It's sacred, and only "somebody who wants to play God" would decide against it. Many of the nurses at Northern General are devoutly religious, and many told me directly that they wouldn't consider giving up on a patient. The question, for them, is not a legitimate one.

3. To some nurses, the technology of medicine demands application. If the machines are there, the logic says, we must use them. Some nurses, however, explicitly reject this attitude. "You have all this medical technology," says one, "but that

6. As Preston says, "Nurses do sometimes petition physicians for restraint, but I have seen meager results. Medical orders are followed and medical drama unfolds at the direction of physicians." Preston, *The Dilemmas of Care*, p. 135.

7. A recent retrospective analysis of CPR, which was essentially invented in its current form in 1960, found the 15 percent figure. A. Patrick Schneider II, Darla J. Nelson, and Donald D. Brown, "In-Hospital Cardiopulmonary Resuscitation: A 30-Year Review," *Journal of the American Board of Family Practice* 6, no. 2 (March-April 1993), pp. 91–101. According to *The Merck Manual*, 13th ed., p. 470: "Breathing and heartbeat have been restored in humans after as long as three h[ours] of resuscitation." For a graphic description of a code, see Preston, *The Dilemmas of Care*, p. 133.

doesn't mean that you have to use it." Then, too, the entire ethos of modern medicine is one of active intervention.

4. For many staff members "the death of a patient is a failure. That's kind of a cliché, but that's true. I mean, if a patient goes down the tubes and dies, the first thing they say to themselves is, 'What did we do wrong?' Maybe they didn't do *anything* wrong, maybe this was this guy's time, you know, his number was up, it's time to go" [Interview]. Zussman quotes a resident as saying, "It's a selfish reason. You know, you try to keep them alive because you're the one that saved this person. I don't know how much it was done because they actually thought they could bring this person back to [being] a viable human being more than we got him to live during his stay in the ICU. In a competitive place where these people pride themselves on being such good doctors, that idea is sometimes prevalent."[8]

New interns in particular seem to suffer: "Half get sick the first time one of their patients dies." And some older doctors as well refuse to give up trying to revive an apparently dead person. In one case, an attending physician, paged when a patient arrested, didn't come immediately. The code team, for some reason, didn't show up ("Didn't show up?" "That's right, no one came"), and when the doctor finally arrived, the patient—a hopeless case to begin with—had been clinically dead for half an hour. The doctor, adamant, ordered that a code be called and started the (hopeless) resuscitation effort [Interview].

5. Sometimes the family is near when the patient arrests. Staff feel awkward standing by and watching someone die while relatives are there. Sometimes, of course, the family members are themselves ambivalent about what should be done.

> There was [a young male patient] . . . nineteen or twenty, and his mother was with him, and he was having some difficulty breathing . . . I just sat down a minute . . . and she started to yell. And we went running in there and we saw that he arrested, so we made the phone call.

8. Zussman, *Intensive Care*, p. 59.

... I would say it was a period of about five minutes that I was resuscitating this young man [before the code team came]. The whole time I was on his chest . . . and the mother was screaming at us to help him, to do him a favor: he would never walk again, he's suffered enough, why resuscitate this young man? . . . I was trying to explain to her that it wasn't my decision. I said to her, you know, "Why don't you go out of the room?" She wouldn't leave the room, and the doctors came . . . We got him back: he was just like he was before.

And her husband came in and she turned around . . . after screaming for half an hour "Why don't you let him die, you're cruel, you're vicious, don't you understand what he's been through?" She turned around and she said to [her husband], "They almost let him die!" [Interview]

In light of such ambivalence, the best rule is: "Do everything to save the patient."

6. A code is a learning experience for the younger physicians, nurses, and medical students. Especially valuable is learning how to pass the endotracheal tube into the lungs, a difficult procedure. The desire to "practice" infuriates some nurses, but it can save lives in the future. For some staff people, the opportunity to practice is good enough reason to code anyone: "Unless the family comes up and says 'we don't want you to do anymore,' then they're gonna go ahead, and bust their butts [trying to CPR]. Everyone's gonna get their chance to defibrillate grandma" [Interview].

7. Finally, continued treatment is often justified on legal grounds. If there is ambiguity about the legal constraints, if the hospital attorney is skeptical, or if anyone is afraid of a lawsuit, treatment may be continued despite the fact that the patient, the family, and the staff want it to stop. Fear of legal entanglements drives many otherwise senseless decisions.

All of these rationales support the imperative to "save the patient." They place the question of resuscitation outside of the nurse's area of immediately felt responsibility. Often rationales are found in a single statement, reinforcing each other:

[A patient] had a massive coronary . . . we got him to the emergency room, then to intensive care. Once you get into that situation, there is nobody who can stop and say, "Let's let him die."

So, he's going to die, and we know he's going to die. And the nicer way to have him die would be by making him comfortable and letting his family be with him. But he's attached to equipment, and when the alarm goes off you have to answer it. When his heart stops beating, you have to start it again . . . It just really goes against my principles [but] that is the job. [Interview]

And, certainly, the great rewards come when some patients are saved. For the nurses involved, this is medical heroism at its best:

I can't tell you what it's like to pump someone's heart and save them. And have [the doctor] go into the family room and say, "Your husband is alive, we've saved your husband."

I did that with a young man who came in, had no hope, he was going to die, that was it. Came in cardiac arrested. We pumped—I did—pumped away, pumped away, and we brought him back. And I went into the family room and said, "Michael's alive." [Interview]

Usually an arresting patient is coded automatically; nobody thinks of letting him or her die. This is probably a good thing. Thinking uses up precious time and distracts nurses and doctors from their unique task of saving people.

Slow Code

A full code, as just described, is an aggressive technique; every effort is made to save the patient's life. But "aggressive" is a relative term, and there are more and less aggressive codes. Sometimes the phone is dialed a bit more slowly, or the code team works a bit less enthusiastically, or maybe they quit after only fifteen minutes instead of after an hour. Some doctors, wanting to avoid the legal and ethical responsibilities of writing a DNR order, may even suggest that a nurse handle the problem of the terminal patient on her own:

[Say] a young staff nurse in charge [with a hopelessly ill patient], maybe there's not a written Do Not Resuscitate order. The intern [on his way out the door] may just, you know, fling over his shoulder, "If Mr. Jones stops breathing, just don't do anything dumb." [Interview]

This puts the doctors in the clear; no one actually said "don't call the code." In one high-mortality unit, there are patients "on every chemical known to God and man," hooked up to all the monitors and machines, eighty years old and hopelessly sick, and "no one will take the responsibility for a DNR order." Feelings from everyone might be clear: the family wants the pain to end, the doctors feel the same, and so do the nurses—but no one will come out and say, "Let's stop." So staff have developed what is called a "slow code." Basically, "we take our time calling for help. We take time getting to the phone" [Interview]. Some nurses won't do this, but ways are found to work around them. Usually, it seems, a consensus has developed.

> Somebody said to us, "This patient needs to be resuscitated," and you know goddamn well that he's probably brain damaged or something, or he's been through 99 arrests already. The family's hurting, he's hurting, and it would just be best to let him pass on. Like I told you, [the staff will] do their own little devices, their slow codes. They take time getting to the phone . . . [It] is all grossly illegal, but they will do that. [Interview]

This cannot always be done. The same nurse continues:

> Still, all in all, at the end, when that patient finally does something death producing, goes into ventricular fibrillation . . . they are compelled to defibrillate the patient . . . If they let them go without ventricular defibrillation, everybody's ass is on the line. [Interview]

Slow codes are an especially interesting case of how an ethical problem can be handled while responsibility for action is muddled. They succeed for at least three reasons:

First, the slow code shifts the problem from medicine, where legal responsibility lies, to nursing. For the most part, it is nurses who "do" it. Their presence on the floor, their discovery of the arrested patient, makes the slow code a possibility for the nursing staff. "Nonrescue" tactics are easiest on night shifts, in single rooms, in restricted areas such as preemie wards (except during baby viewing times), or on private duty.[9] Because it is available especially to nurses, the slow code reflects the nurses' real, if unrecognized, power in the hospital. In some cases a physician may adamantly refuse to let a patient die; but with a slow code, the nurses can circumvent this refusal in a deniable way.

Second, slow codes are based on tacit understandings; their very existence depends on their being unacknowledged, yet silently recognized by the staff. Slow codes are an open secret among hospital personnel—everyone knows of them but no one says much. Nurses know the phrase "slow code." And yet they vary greatly in whether they discuss such things with peers. In some quarters, it seemed, it was done but never discussed. Silence protects the notion that slow codes don't really happen, at least not officially. Therefore, they are very hard to stop.[10]

Third, slow codes are inherently ambiguous. It's ambiguous that anything has been done (how fast should one get to the phone?) or that anyone definite has done it. The ambiguity of action is tremendous here, and ambiguity allows things to happen without anyone having caused it. Perhaps it was an event, but an organizational one.

Slow codes work because every step in saving a life involves an action, and every action can be performed without zest. At each step, from the patient's arresting to the implementation of heroic measures, nurses and doctors can move slowly or stop. Perhaps at first no one sees the patient; no one calls the code; they go slowly to call it; when the doctors arrive, things are handled casually; and so on. At no point was an explicit decision made to let this patient die. Responsibility then is deniable. Perhaps, as philosopher Andrew Jameton suggests, this is ethically wrong: "The practice of slow codes is vastly inferior, ethically and procedurally, to openly discussing such decisions and charting them in the case record. Slow codes usually indicate unclarity about goals of treatment, lack of communication

9. See also Glaser and Strauss, *Awareness of Dying*, pp. 219–220.
10. See Daniel F. Chambliss, "Slow Codes and Ambiguous Euthanasia," paper presented at the annual meeting of the Law and Society Association, Madison, Wisconsin, June 1989.

among staff, unwillingness to acknowledge a terminal prognosis, or an attempt to create a charade of all-out effort for the
family and the law."[11] But they are conducted, nevertheless.

In the hospital, then, choices can be made by *not* acting
decisively. A patient can be left on a respirator, and that's "no
decision." Or an operation can be postponed; if the patient
dies, perhaps a "judgment error" was made, but that's not euthanasia. A woman gives birth to a grossly deformed infant,
and she delays consenting to the needed treatment until the
infant dies on its own. In all these cases—and the slow code is
in some ways a prototype of them—decisions are made by not
acting quickly. The claim can then be that no decision in fact
was made, and that responsibility for the death lies somewhere
else.

Such practices, however, do change over time. It is my
clear impression that between 1979, when I began studying
hospitals, and 1990, when the fieldwork for this book ended,
slow codes decreased in frequency. This probably happened
because of the nationwide acceptance of guidelines for Do Not
Resuscitate policies. With those guidelines, doctors were explicitly allowed to write DNR orders; the responsibility for the
decision was clear, officially approved procedures could be ad-
hered to, and all parties were legally protected. In this case the
introduction of formal ethics, along with review committees,
standards of decision making, and a clarified language for discussion of cases has truly made a difference. It has eliminated
the need for the subterfuges of which slow codes are only a
particularly sharp example. As it became clear that physicians
could—and would—sign DNR orders, it seems the incentive
for slow codes has declined sharply.

Stopping Treatments
To keep acutely ill patients alive, staff perform a broad array of
treatments. Ceasing or limiting these treatments may increase a
patient's likelihood of dying soon. Then again, it may not matter much, as Zussman suggests was the case at his sites: "But
the difference in the death rate of those patients for whom

11. Jameton, *Nursing Practice*, p. 233.

treatment was in fact limited is only slightly higher than the death rate among those patients for whom limiting treatment was discussed but decided against (92 percent compared to 86 percent at Outerboro, 78 percent compared to 71 percent at Countryside), statistically insignificant differences."[12] Treatments, therefore, may be discontinued as "futile."

"Discontinuing treatment" can mean many things. Terminal cancer patients may decline a last desperate round of chemotherapy, or one more pointless, mutilating operation. A nurse, seeing a hopeless patient, may stop giving medications

> . . . because the patient's going to die, and no one knows you didn't do this or you didn't do that. You can falsify . . . on [the] . . . med sheet, very easily, by saying you gave the med and didn't give it. [Interview]

Antibiotic medications can be stopped, with the result that an immuno-compromised patient (one very susceptible to infection, perhaps because of leukemia or AIDS) will often contract pneumonia or septicemia and die quickly. Stopping kidney dialysis will lead to uremic poisoning and death.[13] These are ambiguous forms of "letting die." Nurses sometimes complain about the "active-passive euthanasia bit, if there's a difference," as one says. She complains of an order to stop antibiotics, so the patient takes days to die. Why not just directly give morphine to kill the patient less painfully?

"Do Not Resuscitate": The Formal Order
"Do Not Resuscitate" ("DNR") is a formal order, written on the patient's chart, which indicates that if the patient arrests no attempt will be made at resuscitation. DNR orders are quite common. In a large hospital, on any particular day a number of patients (perhaps a dozen, say) will be "DNR" or "No Code." DNR orders have been given ever since resuscitation techniques became available, but they were subject to major policy changes during the 1980s. At the beginning of the decade, the

---

12. Zussman, *Intensive Care*, p. 131.

13. See Renée C. Fox and Judith P. Swazey, *The Courage to Fail*, rev. ed. (Chicago: University of Chicago Press, 1978), on kidney dialysis.

legal status of DNR orders was doubtful, so many physicians avoided writing them for fear of legal trouble. The "slow code" was a more common means of allowing death without writing a formal order. But in the late 1980s, the Joint Commission on Accredition of Health Care Organizations mandated that all hospitals in the United States have an official policy. This gave institutional legitimacy to the DNR (or No Code) decision. What had once been the private decision of those at the bedside had become the institutional decision of the organization and was officially recognized.[14] This development works to the benefit of nurses.

> Nursing staff is really verbal about DNRs, because we're with the patient the most. We see what those poor bastards go through. Seriously, when someone's been resuscitated nine or ten times and their chest looks like raw meat, they've been fried from being defibrillated, they've had their chest pumped on, they've got a flat chest because their ribs are no more connected to their sternum . . . You know this guy doesn't have a chance in hell. I mean, he's already blown out, squash, herniated his brain, he doesn't have any spontaneous respirations, he's flat EEGs. You take care of him for eight hours, you know that this person is not viable, and you feel for him and you feel for the family . . . When you're resuscitating somebody and they get no response going into the code for an hour, and now has no EKG, no heart tracing, pupils are blown, fixed, no spontaneous respiration, blood gases are out in the ozone . . . you are the one that's going to turn to the resident and say, "Don't you think this is about it, don't you think we should call this?" [Interview]

So nurses find themselves asking for a formal DNR order to end the struggle. With a written order, or at least "an explicit verbal order," the issue of whether to let the patient die or not is "redefined as a nonproblem," as one nurse says; the ethical problem is transposed into a medical one, and medicine is the doctors' province.

At the same time, executing a DNR order is most difficult for the nurses, who must stand by and do nothing when the

---

14. Information came directly to me in a letter from the Joint Commission on Accreditation of Health Care Organizations; see also Rothman, *Strangers at the Bedside*.

patient arrests. Although the legal or role responsibility may lie elsewhere, the nurse is organizationally responsible for carrying out the "no code." The nurse must sit and watch the patient turn blue, and listen to the patient gurgle, drowning in his or her own juices.

Officially, physicians are responsible for signing DNR orders. Often, though, according to nurses, the responsibility is dodged:

> They don't do it. They won't write "DNR." So we write "DNR per verbal order of." We say, do you want this patient to be DNR? If they say "yes," we go write this in the chart. Basically, they want to keep their hands and their noses clean. [Interview]

The doctors, claim nurses, stay away from the floor, or are too busy, or just give an indication they *think* a DNR would be good. But often they won't write it down, a nurse says. A written order will make the clear responsibility fall to the doctor, and, say nurses, "it'll be easier for us." But the doctors, for their part—especially the young ones, interns and residents—feel bad about DNRs and resist "staking" a patient (letting a patient die), so they will sometimes try to get the family to say, "Let him go," or some such. In general, it seems that everyone involved with a DNR decision has some desire to sidestep responsibility for this awesome decision. Families may rather have the doctors, the "experts," decide; and staff will argue that families should make the decision themselves.

Despite the legal placement of responsibility with the physician, there seems in practice to be a broader institutionalization of the decision; there seems to be some tendency to share the burden among the staff. One nurse says that

> nobody will take responsibility for saying, "I am the one that said this patient is DNR." . . . Half the time we don't know where it comes from. We just know that that's the consensus of opinion. It's a consensus-of-opinion order. DNR. It's a group order. [Interview]

Some hospitals have more formal mechanisms for "corporatizing" ethically difficult choices. In the two large teaching hospitals I studied, certain physicians, nurses, and administrators are known to be professionally interested in ethical problems. They are editors of journals on the subject, widely read authors on ethical problems in health care, and speakers much in demand on these issues. These in-house experts, who sometimes advocate controversial positions, are often consulted for advice on life-terminating actions. At Northern General, there was an official ethics committee available for consultation by physicians unsure of what to do. Southwestern Regional Hospital also had a system of "ethics consultations" available. The guidelines outline how decisions should be made—recognizing that the family's wishes should be respected, for instance, or that patient autonomy should be maintained. Guidelines provide support to the concerned staff person. At the same time, committees and guidelines can help to psychologically unburden the individual staff member faced with the dilemmas discussed. People are afraid of "playing God"; guidelines remind them that they are not God. There are other people involved, and the possibilities are not limitless. In ethical dilemmas where there is no single right answer, guidelines help us believe that at least we pick the preferable answer; and they fortify the belief that the decision comes not from an individual but from the group.

Withdrawal of Ventilator Support
A DNR order states that a particular patient whose breathing and circulation fails should not be revived. But some patients are revived, only to become dependent on the mechanical breathing machine (called either a "ventilator" or "respirator") which pumps air into the lungs. To survive, a patient must eventually be "weaned" off the ventilator, so that the lungs regain their natural function. Normally, this takes place within a few days. But some patients, seriously ill, stay on the respirator for a longer time, which makes weaning more difficult. The lungs lose their elasticity, the body becomes dependent on the high concentrations of oxygen pumped in, and the patient becomes "respirator dependent." Or lungs, hopelessly weakened by disease (for instance, emphysema), haven't the strength to breathe without help. And so this patient, too, is respirator dependent.

"At this stage," say Glaser and Strauss, "nurses invariably

favor letting the patient die, realizing, of course, that they do not actually have to 'pull the cord.'"[15] They can allow the patient to die through the gradual, or even immediate, removal of the patient from the ventilator. The machines are adjustable in various ways (for oxygen mixture, volume delivered, air pressure, etc.), and the adjustments affect the patient's condition. Adjustments can be manipulated so as to allow a patient to die, but in such a way that no active intervention in nature's course was taken. Withdrawal of the highly artificial, even invasive, breathing support system is hardly active "euthanasia."

> You don't shut off the respirator, per se, OK, you slow it down. We used to wean somebody, put them on "blow-by," which means to put them on oxygen, so maybe they would be able to breathe for themselves for half an hour and then they would die. [Interview]

This technique allows several people to be involved, but no one person does "it." One nurse told me of a doctor who got a respiratory therapist (RT) to turn down a patient's respirator a little; and then, a few days later, down again, and so on; and one day the patient died. The RT had assumed that the doctor knew best and that the patient was in fact improving. (But other nurses say such a thing couldn't be true; the RT would know.) The physician never had to deal face-to-face with the consequences of his order, though he had certainly made the decision.[16] Weaning in this way is an attempt to end things by returning the patient to a pretreatment state. "He's in God's hands now," seems to be the feeling.

Less ambiguous is the actual disconnection of the respirator from a dependent patient. The lay public calls this "pulling the plug." In this process the patient will usually be "extubated"—the endotracheal tube is removed—and the machine taken away. In such cases, death is projected as almost inevitable, and it becomes more obvious that a decision has been made to let the patient die. Responsibility is more definite.

15. Glaser and Strauss, *Awareness of Dying*, p. 198.

16. For another case of "euthanasia by ventilation adjustment," see Preston, *The Dilemmas of Care*, pp. 183–184.

One such case, involving a newborn infant, is recorded in my interview notes, and I quote them here at length:

> Baby D——, in Newborn Unit: been here 5 months. Parents are a 14-year-old girl and 19-year-old man. Baby was responsive, would look at you, but no hope of surviving off the ventilator, lungs totally wrecked.
>
> Mother's parents were supportive of parents' decision to let the child go; father's parents were "hoping for a miracle" (as it said in nursing notes). Finally parents were told that "you have to make this decision, you're the ones who have to live with it," and they eventually decided to let her go. They began visiting more, holding the baby, talking to it, asking [the head nurse] questions.
>
> The night before [the ventilator would be dc'd], the head nurse and the parents were awake all night; so was the doctor, all thinking about it. They came in that morning, it had been planned for 8:00 A.M., but they had to wait until 2 o'clock that afternoon ("that was terrible," said one nurse), because the doctors kept delaying, perhaps because other people were in the unit.
>
> [The head nurse] and the (female) doctor did it. When they disconnected the ventilator, the baby's eyes widened in surprise, she flailed about for a minute; she had been restrained, they untied her. They had given her some morphine IM [intramuscular, an injection]; they were unable to start an IV, all the veins were blown, so the IM morphine, less effective, had to be used. [The head nurse] held it close, the infant flailed some more and began gasping. It took about fifteen minutes, which is fairly quick. [Interviews]

Another nurse comments on her feelings when she handled a similar case:

> They said her respirator was to be dc'd [disconnected] and, uh, the respiratory therapist and myself dc'd, and she died immediately . . . [I had] never [done] anything quite that, uh, quite that cut and dried . . . It just felt very, uh, I felt very godly or something . . . like I have these—this power of life and death and absolutely no right. And I think I was angry with the medi-

cal profession for allowing me to be the one to have to make
this kind of—or *do* this kind of thing. [Interview]

This nurse was irritated that the responsibility was in her
hands; she would rather the doctors disconnected the respirator. She was bothered, too, that she had to do it so directly:

> I was just annoyed that it was asked of me . . . when all the
> other nurses had very discreet and subtle ways of doing these
> things. [Interview]

No one person, the nurse felt, should have to do *this*.
There are organizational techniques for ceasing support which
protect discrete individuals, especially those without the legal
responsibility. It should be an organizational or collective act.

Indeed, the society as a whole has become a background
participant to such decisions since the famous Karen Ann
Quinlan case of the late 1970s. Quinlan was a young woman
who, under the influence of alcohol and perhaps other drugs,
slipped into an irreversible coma. Her parents sought, after it
became apparent that their daughter would never recover, to
have Karen Ann disconnected from the respirator which kept
her alive. Against the wishes of the doctors and the hospital,
who feared legal repercussions, they wanted to "pull the plug."
The New Jersey Supreme Court ruled that disconnection
would be allowed. As the court's opinion said:

> If . . . there is no reasonable possibility of Karen's ever emerging
> from her present comatose condition to a cognitive, sapient
> state, the present life-support system may be withdrawn and
> said action shall be without any civil or criminal liability . . . We
> do not intend to be understood as implying that a proceeding
> for judicial declaratory relief is necessarily required for the im-
> plementation of comparable decisions in the field of medical
> practice.

Together with the later (1990) U.S. Supreme Court decision in the case of Nancy Cruzan, this decision reshaped DNR
policy in America.[17]

17. The Supreme Court of New Jersey, "In the Matter of Karen Quinlan,"
355.2d 647 (1976); *Cruzan v. Director*, Missouri Dept. of Health, et al., 58USLW
4916 (US, June 25, 1990).

A nurse at Northern General commented:

> I remember before Karen Ann Quinlan, they turned off the
> respirators [occasionally] . . . now they do that a lot more often.
> Usually you can get the private doctors to go in and do it . . .
> Maybe after you've practiced [medicine] 25 years [you can say]
> . . . "I really don't think this person is going to make it." And
> they pull it . . . take out the tubes, turn off the respirator.
> [Interview]

And yet what is new is not disconnecting respirators but
all the publicity and legal sanctions for it. As Peggy Anderson
said in her book *Nurse:*

> I think the [Quinlan] case was blown far out of proportion . . .
> decisions are made every day to let patients go when lifesaving
> measures are no longer deemed appropriate.[18]

Such disconnections are in fact quite a matter of course, and
the Quinlan case is only notable because it went to court and
attracted tremendous publicity. Still, it has provided a reference point for many medical workers: first, that the legal system does occasionally intervene, and things could get nasty;
and second, that courts may allow for discontinuation of support. *Quinlan* marked the point at which the courts became a
full-fledged player in medical-ethical decisions, and the publicity around the case reminded health care workers that their
decisions were no longer inviolably private. In this respect
Quinlan profoundly reshaped the context of life-and-death decisions.

The adjustment or disconnection of a ventilator are two
ways in which support can be withdrawn to let a patient die.
At other times, as I have mentioned earlier in this chapter,
kidney dialysis is stopped, so the patient succumbs to uremic
poisoning; or necessary medication such as antibiotics are withdrawn, so that infection sets in and the patient dies relatively
quickly from, say, pneumonia. When this is done, no one actually makes a decision to kill the patient. They just apply the
"active-passive euthanasia bit." The "bit" distinguishes the passive withdrawal of support from active homicide. The patient

18. Anderson, *Nurse,* p. 68.

lingers when passive methods are used, so some people argue that active euthanasia is thus better. But there are clear advantages to withdrawal of support. Legally, it seems somewhat accepted, as in the Quinlan case. And it diffuses responsibility among a large group of people: no one person actually lets the patient die.

Discretionary Use of Medications
There is one more common technique for managing death, one which clearly poses the dilemma of caring for a patient versus preserving life. This technique is the heavy use of drugs, especially opiates, to control intractable pain. Nurses typically administer such drugs. Often a physician will write an order that may say, "10 mg. of morphine sulfate 2 hrs PRN"—that is, every two hours, as needed. This "PRN"—as needed—is crucial. For what if a patient's pain is truly intractable and repeated full dosages are needed? Continuing heavy doses of opiates (called "snowing" in hospital slang) suppresses the central nervous system, slows breathing, and can eventually cause death.[19]

So the nurse's effort to free the patient from pain conflicts directly with her fear of killing the patient through treatment.

We had two or three patients, and they were terminally ill with cancer. We would give the patients, every two or three hours around the clock toward the end, morphine sulphate, intramuscular.

I was really worried about giving them a morphine injection because the morphine depresses the respiration. I thought, well, is this injection going to do them in?

If I don't give the injection, they will linger on longer, but they might also have more pain. If I do give the injection, the end result of death is going to occur faster. Am I playing God? [Interview]

Or:

We had a 17-year-old boy dying of Crohn's disease . . . supposed to get 10 mg. of morphine every hour. But morphine comes in

19. See also Glaser and Strauss, *Awareness of Dying*, pp. 197–198.

ampules of 15. Do I waste the rest, given that he needs more for the pain? I gave him the 15: strictly illegal, I was helping kill him. [Interview]

The nurse who "snows" such a patient can ease her anxiety by focusing on *care:*

Well, we are making the patient really comfortable. But I still think it bothers me a lot. I turn my thinking around from "I'm killing this person" to "I'm making them more comfortable." [Interview]

Or she can point to the patient's condition. A diagnosis of cancer, for instance, seems to legitimate the unlimited use of drugs. It lets the nurse feel that it's acceptable to give the medication, even if the dosage may cause the patient to arrest. A cancer diagnosis, it seems, is a justification as well as a reason to use drugs to their utmost.

Other coping mechanisms are less purely psychological. Nurses can share their responsibility:

The patient was going to die, was in bad shape, and the nurses more or less got together . . . They continued giving the [morphine] shots, but what they did was take turns giving them . . . so that no one would feel that they were really [giving the final injection]. [Interview]

The responsibility of each nurse is thus diffused among the group. This way, if their fear that "it'll be after *my* shot" comes true, the act was committed by the group.

But sometimes turns aren't taken; sometimes nurses know what has occurred and who did it:

R.K. [a nurse] said that she had given lots of morphine to an old man, keeping him out of pain. He had made it clear, and his family had too, that he wanted "a dignified death." She said, "In effect, I was killing him, and I don't feel bad about it." She was incredibly straightforward. [Field Notes]

There are still more active forms of euthanasia than those discussed here. Injections of Valium or potassium chloride could be given, or food or water could be withheld.[20] These pose obvious ethical and psychological problems. Giving a fatal injection is an unambiguous act, and a single person does it; the organization in no sense does it, and so it clearly falls within the individual actor's circle of responsibility. When I have heard such acts discussed among nurses, no one spoke of a doctor's orders, or blamed the family's wishes, or mentioned guidelines. Guidelines don't seem to cover here.

Unfortunately, the danger of legal prosecution keeps people from telling what they know of active euthanasia. As any newspaper writer could attest, when prosecutors start demanding to know your sources, the sources dry up. So almost all we have for confessional literature on active euthanasia are anonymous articles[21] and books delivered under pseudonyms.[22] On the rare occasion that an attempt at euthanasia comes into the open, the public is surprised and alarmed. Most people seem to think that euthanasia, in its various forms, is either new or rare, whereas people familiar with hospitals suggest that it is neither. In 1991, James Rachels, a well-known medical ethicist who teaches at the University of Alabama, said in a lecture at the University of Tennessee at Chattanooga that he could find only three instances in U.S. history in which a physician was charged with murder in a euthanasia case. These occurred in 1950 (via the injection of an air bubble), 1974 (by potassium chloride), and 1988 (method unspecified). And then one could add the "doctor-assisted suicides" of Dr. Jack Kevorkian, as mentioned earlier, which began in 1990. Occasionally a case surfaces involving nurses, and these attract tremendous amounts of publicity, but criminal convictions seem to be very unusual. Regardless, active euthanasia is probably rare, since passive forms are so available. As we have seen, they are legally

20. Regarding injections, see Robert M. Veatch, *Death, Dying, and the Biological Revolution* (New Haven: Yale University Press, 1976), chap. 3; regarding withholding nutrition, see Raymond S. Duff and A. G. M. Campbell, "Moral and Ethical Dilemmas in the Special Care Nursery," *New England Journal of Medicine* 289, October 25, 1973.

21. For two examples, see Terry Daniels, "The Nurse's Tale," *New York*, April 30, 1979, pp. 37–41; and Dr. X, "I Pulled the Plug," *Family Health* (July/August 1980), pp. 30–32.

22. For instance, see Anderson, *Nurse*.

ambiguous (is a slow code legal?), and they often disperse responsibility over a number of people.

Still, sometimes a willing informant speaks about active euthanasia. In 1979, I recorded the following in my field notes. The speaker was a nurse whom I did not know well and whose last name I didn't know. After writing my doctoral dissertation, from which the following was deleted for legal reasons, I took my notes and destroyed what little identifying information I then had. Now I retain only this excerpt:

> "I'm in favor of euthanasia," [a nurse] said. People who aren't "haven't seen enough suffering" and don't know how bad the "quality of life" can be.
>
> When she was a new grad, there was a lady [a patient] with metastasized cancer all over—had had everything out—bladder, bowel, esophagus, lungs, stomach. Doc called [this nurse] into the room, said to fill a syringe with Valium; she gave it to him. He drew the curtains around them and the bed and gave the pt a shot of Valium in the femoral artery, putting her to sleep; killing her.
>
> The doc turned to ——, who was crying, and said, "I'm sorry." She said he shouldn't apologize, that she was glad he did it. [Field Notes]

THE DIFFUSION OF RESPONSIBILITY

In all of these cases described here save the last, responsibility is diffused away from individuals and to the hospital and to its customs. This happens in trivial matters as well, in a variety of ways. Sometimes hospital policies are mentioned. When a nurse tells a noisy family to leave, she blames the visitation policy; when a patient wants to see his chart and the nurse refuses to show it, she cites regulations: "Patients look at charts only upon discharge and in the presence of a physician." ("When are such policies used?" I asked one nurse. "When we think they are right," she replied. She added that a "formal" tone of voice emphasized the impersonal nature of the rule.) Regulations can be quoted. In one instance, I saw a nurse spot a patient smoking (this is against rules in many areas). Rather than speaking directly to the patient, the nurse went to her

station, turned on the PA system and said, "Hospital regulations prohibit the use of smoking materials." The nurse thus
doubly separated herself from speaking to the patient personally, first by the use of the electronic PA system, and second
by a mechanical recitation of a relevant rule. On some floors,
guidelines ("Guidelines for priority discharge," "Guidelines for
confidentiality") are posted, as much to support the nurses as
to remind them that rules are to be followed. To remind doctors of their duty, a sign on the wall of the staff room reads:
"Do Not Resuscitate orders must be written in full."

Besides hospital regulations, "Doctor's orders" can remove
a sense of liability from the nurse. Typically, orders are followed, even if reluctantly. Although the nurse has a legal responsibility to refuse an order that she believes to be harmful
to the patient, written or spoken orders provide her the most
tangible and authoritative source of direction. Doctor's orders
can diminish a nurse's sense of responsibility; wishful thinking
aside, nurses are clearly subordinates:

> [T]he physician viewed the nurse's role in the hospital and in
> the care of patients as primarily one of carrying out his orders,
> and reporting the patient's progress to him. Nurses reiterated
> this viewpoint.[23]

The doctor's orders can protect the nurse from responsibility.
There are "medical decisions" best made by the physician; indeed, through orders, an ethical decision can be transformed
into a medical or technical one. A written order, in particular,
separates nurses from responsibility for what they do in several
ways:[24] (1) It physically separates the physician who gives it
from the nurse who follows it. This makes the interaction less
subordinating for the nurse; she submits to the order on paper, not to the person of the doctor. (2) In writing, the order
becomes part of the hospital authority. It's on a form, in the
chart, part of the record. The decision becomes reified, a real
thing, and everyone is then somehow committed to it. (3) The

23. Raymond S. Duff and August B. Hollingshead, *Sickness and Society* (New
York: Harper & Row, 1968), p. 217.
24. For an excellent discussion, see Rose Laub Coser, *Life in the Ward* (East
Lansing: Michigan State University Press, 1962), pp. 24–25.

order can then be responded to as part of a professional task, part of "being a nurse." It is no longer a command from one person to another; it is a professional communication.

Thus, medical orders, like formal regulations, remove personal considerations and allow nurses to describe their actions as organizationally required instead of personally motivated. In keeping with this, nurses may try to define their relationship with doctors as a "legal" one, as Rose Coser suggests:

> By her insistence on rules and her refusal to be considered a "servant" who has to do the doctor's "dirty work," the nurse is emphasizing that hospital organization is based on a "legal order" in which the authority and responsibility of the members are defined and limited, rather than on a "traditional order" where the one who obeys orders is "subordinate with his total personality."[25]

The nurse, then, is an employee of the hospital, subject to the control of administrators and their rules. And she takes orders from physicians, with their greater power, prestige, and knowledge as well as their traditional male dominance. Recognizing this state of affairs can protect her from responsibility. The claim that one is weak, that someone else is in charge, allows the nurse to escape personal criticism for her actions, however she personally feels about them.

Other factors can also diffuse a nurse's sense of personal responsibility. In the early 1960s social psychologists Bibb Latané and John Darley argued that the more people present at a scene, the less any one of them will feel responsible for what happens.[26] This hypothesis suggests that the larger an organization, the less likely any member is to feel responsible for its actions. The contemporary medical center is clearly a large organization, offering many other potential centers of responsibility. The presence of experts may mean the moral abdication of those who are not experts. People may assume that the experts know best, and that if the experts don't do something it probably doesn't need doing. Hospitals include committees

25. Ibid., p. 26.
26. Bibb Latané and John M. Darley, *The Unresponsive Bystander: Why Doesn't He Help?* (Englewood Cliffs, NJ: Prentice-Hall, 1970).

of experts on various subjects, who issue reports and guidelines and statements. So ethical problems may be ignored by a nurse, not because she can't deal with them but, in a sense, because too many other people can. It's easy here to be overwhelmed by both the sheer number of other people and by their apparent expertise. The individual nurse near the bottom of the hierarchy may ask, What can my opinion be worth?

Finally, perhaps the very weight of a hospital's history can break up belief in individual responsibility. Old hospitals are permeated by tradition, a tradition written down in procedures and rules, made concrete in vast amounts of expensive equipment, and animated in the persons of veteran staff members. This "embodied" tradition means that the hospital as an organization has habits, has usual ways of doing things. It is, in March and Olsen's phrase, a collection of "solutions looking for problems."[27] CAT scanners, the expensive machines for taking three-dimensional X-rays, may be used more often than necessary to justify the expense of having bought them; the easy availability of elaborate diagnostic tests almost seems to tempt physicians to use them. A kind of "technological imperative" can take hold. In a similar way, old habits, embodied in people, may run the hospital, whether or not they are still appropriate. So again, no single person feels that they make decisions; instead, they say, "This is the way things are done here."

So in multiple ways the organization presents opportunities for the setting aside of individual responsibility. It provides a setting for individual action—in this case, a setting that is large, technological, dense with expertise, hierarchical, and roughly fragmented. For the individual nurse, this means that the organization allows her to do things that she may believe wrong, in the belief that "that's how things work," "others know better than I," or "it's a big place so how can I know the whole story?" There are opportunities for the nurse to be ignorant of what is happening with a patient (the patient can be hidden, physically and socially), and she can turn her eyes to other tasks, of which she has many. As Glaser and Strauss

---

27. James G. March and Johann Olsen, *Ambiguity and Choice in Organizations* (Bergen: Universitet Forlaget, 1976), passim.

say, "Nurses also take advantage of the hospital organization when they avoid spending time with the patient by doing some other work, by spending time with other patients, or by charting back at the nursing station."[28] These same opportunities let the nurse protect herself from the encroachments of the hospital and the problems she finds in it; they let her feel that decisions are out of her hands, and that her own sense of ethics is safe even while she does things she may believe to be wrong.

Christopher Stone, in writing about problems of responsibility in business corporations, points to the difficulty in preventing a diffusion of responsibility in situations like this:

> As corporations increase in size, and production processes become more complex, and more and more persons (and machines) have a hand in the finished product, it is increasingly difficult to locate responsibility on any one particular individual *for that end product:* the defective car or the building that collapses.[29]

As labor is divided, so too is responsibility. An ethical problem—a patient who refuses blood transfusions, or a patient who wants to die despite attempts to save him—can be wheeled from place to place, literally coming in one door and going out the other. This is, after all, part of what is implied in a division of labor: work is divided up, and responsibility is scattered. As C. Wright Mills says: "In a world dominated by a vast system of abstractions, managers may become cold with principle and do what local and immediate masters of men could never do . . . The social control of the system is such that irresponsibility is organized into it."[30]

Paradoxically, as we have seen, these very features that are opportunities for denying responsibility are also, at the same time, opportunities to take responsibility. The very size of the hospital, the very elaborateness of the division of labor there, mean that not only can problems be hidden but that aggressive

28. Glaser and Strauss, *Awareness of Dying*, p. 57.

29. Christopher Stone, *Where the Law Ends* (New York: Harper & Row, 1976), p. 190.

30. C. Wright Mills, *White Collar* (London: Oxford University Press, 1951), pp. 110–111.

action can be taken, vast discretion exercised, awesome choices can be made, and yet all of it remain invisible. But even when such choices are made, as in the choice to let a patient die, the usual effect of the staff's handling of death is to reinforce in their minds the place of the organization itself as the effective moral actor.

Conclusion

This book has presented a view of the meaning of morality inside large organizations (hospitals) as experienced by people who work there (nurses). Moral and ethical challenges in nursing, we have now seen, are systemic features of the contemporary hospital; they are a normal part of its operations rather than external or accidental. The organization's structure determines both what are seen as problems and how those problems are managed.

My argument has been developed as a series of themes:

1. *Routinization creates a different sense of what is "normal" in the hospital.* The nurse's daily reality differs from that of the layperson, since she has routinized many things that the rest of us would experience as frightening or horrible. Much that we would see as difficult she finds normal, so she faces moral issues from a different baseline. Most nursing issues never reach an ethics committee or spark a formal debate; instead, they are handled in routine ways. Nurses for the most part accept this routine and actively protect it when chaos threatens to challenge the stable order of hospital life (see Chaps. 1 and 2).

2. *The nurse's role in the hospital is shaped by multiple, sometimes contradictory, imperatives.* The nurse is a paid employee of the hospital, but she is more than that. She is actively encouraged to be, simultaneously, a caring person, a committed professional, and a loyal subordinate. Obviously, these components of her role frequently conflict with each other (Chap. 3).

3. *Ethical problems in nursing primarily reflect conflict between nurses and other constituencies in the hospital.* In this sense, the

"shape" of an organization, especially its division of labor, creates conflicts. When these conflicts are described in moral terminology, they become "ethical problems" for the staff. Of course, nurses do have personal dilemmas, in which they can't decide the right thing to do. But more often they face political difficulties in dealing with physicians, administrators, and others, which they experience as moral conflicts. More generally, it seems that the idea of "dilemmas," so central to our usual language of ethics, is appropriate primarily for actors who are relatively autonomous or powerful. Subordinates (such as nurses, or most people) are less concerned with dilemmas than with practical difficulties of working with, or under, other people. The flourishing of medical ethics debates from the late 1960s through the 1980s resulted in part from the fragmentation of the medical profession's monopoly over decision making; as multiple groups join the debate, each with its own agenda, "ethics problems" multiply as well (Chap. 4).

4. *The objectification of patients, and their resistance to objectification, produces a special set of ethical problems for the staff.* Again, what are labeled ethical problems are more accurately described as power conflicts. The objectivity of scientific medicine holds the possibility of objectification of patients—that is, of treating them purely as objects. Patients will resist being treated as objects, thus presenting the staff with questions of who has the power to define the situation and make decisions. These conflicts result not from scientific objectivity per se but from the unilateral exercise of power in imposing this view on patients. Again, these problems result neither from the obstreperousness of particular patients nor from the scientific ethos of modern medicine alone, but from the power conflict between staff and patients over whose view of disease will take precedence (Chap. 5).

5. *Even in the management of death, the organization remains the effective moral actor.* Until recently, when reproductive technology questions (surrogate motherhood, e.g.) have come to the fore, the most widely discussed issues in bioethics have been those regarding terminally ill patients, such as Karen Ann Quinlan. Such cases occur frequently in large hospitals, and the routines both of keeping the patient alive or of letting her die are handled organizationally. The work is shared

among staff members. The attending physician retains formal responsibility for these decisions (and this was clarified during the 1980s), but in a wide array of cases actions are designed so that no one person is uniquely responsible for the death (Chap. 6).

In sum, *ethical problems in health care are inseparable from the organizational and social settings in which they arise.* Such problems are not random or isolated failures of the system; they are in fact often fundamental, if unintended, products of that system.

The problems nurses face are not logical quandaries, they are political conflicts; not random events but recurring patterns; not psychological "dilemmas" but political conflicts; and they are decided not by the most thoughtful or educated person but by the most powerful. And increasingly that "most powerful person" is not even a human being. It is, instead, an organization or an entire health care system.

Implications

My argument has implications for ethicists, for nurses, and for sociologists; it also may suggest something about the respective places of drama and routine in everyday life.

For the study and practice of biomedical ethics, the implications are far-reaching. At the risk of repeating myself, they are:

1. The assumption of relatively autonomous decision makers is simply unrealistic. Most of us work in organizations, and most decisions of consequence are made in organizational settings and are not localizable to an individual person.

2. People work in organizational and professional roles and settings, and these shape their behavior; ethical decisions are not made in some hypothetical "free choice zone." Nurses, for instance, *by definition* work with other people: a nurse must have patients to be a nurse; to work in a hospital, she must work in some particular hospital, with its own customs and constraints. She works under professional obligations and with real peers who pressure her, need her support, and ask her help. Some of her actions—a nighttime slow code, for instance—are possible only because of the structure of her work:

the absence of the family or physicians, the incompetence of the patient, or the ambiguity of time. To pretend that someone is good or bad apart from settings which allow or prevent their acting is abstraction in the worst sense and pragmatically foolish. It's fine to say, for instance, that doctors should care for each patient as a unique human being, but it won't happen as long as residents see forty to fifty patients a day.

3. Power is a critical variable in determining what will be seen as an ethical problem, in how public the debate becomes, and in the solution reached.

4. Many of the potential "great issues" of medical ethics have been routinized out of existence, for instance, when to turn attention to health (after people are sick); how to understand illness (as a pathophysiological event); and where to treat sick people (in a hospital). Recently, the question of how to pay for health care was raised for new consideration, but only because the current arrangements are bankrupting some powerful businesses. And President Clinton's plan of 1994 didn't even address all the other questions.

5. Finally, since the great problems of health care are structural and not the result of poor reasoning, the solutions cannot be created by increasing education, holding ethics seminars, or (alas) writing books. In overestimating the good effects of such cognitive solutions, perhaps we academics are all alike.

Traditional humanistic ethics has not yet been equipped to draw such conclusions as these on its own. For one thing, ethicists are predominantly theologians or philosophers, not social scientists. They also have tended to address bioethical concerns which have been noticed by participants; their debates are in that sense narrowly selected. Hospital ethics committees discuss problems brought to them—a very small, nonrandom sample of events in health care. This is a significant flaw.

But I don't want to denigrate the tremendous contribution the bioethics movement has made in drawing attention to major issues, in supporting the legitimacy of public debate, and in asserting patients' rights in health care. Ethicists have been instrumental in protecting research subjects, in lobbying for

Living Will and "advance directives" legislation, and in generally focusing attention on the moral dimension of health care. My argument here is intended not as an attack on those efforts but rather as a contribution to them.

Ethics should change its approach; for nursing, the crucial task is more a matter of regaining confidence in its own validity. The facts are these:

1. Nurses are not the lowest people in the hospital hierarchy, but they are clearly subordinates: often ignored, shown little respect, and generally undervalued. They carry out vital work and are typically not recognized or rewarded for that. Much of their work is of low visibility and of little dramatic potential. In this their situation is typical of that of many women.

2. This is not to say that nurses are morally better than doctors or anyone else. They are fundamentally employees in a helping profession. Their self-description as "patient advocates" is as much ideology as objective description.

3. For nursing especially, politics and ethics are intertwined. For nurses to do good, they must have the *power* to do good; currently, many nurses feel they aren't given that power. This accounts for their experience that ethical problems are less dilemmas of conscience than practical troubles with actually doing what they feel is right.

4. But nurses don't want to "play God"; they are not seeking the responsibility of making big decisions by themselves. Most often, I think, they are just trying to do what they see as their proper job and to get the resources to do that job.

For nursing as a profession, the great moral danger would be for nursing to lose its own center and to subordinate itself to the goals and values of medicine—seeking medicine's prestige, or hoping to borrow by association some of its respect. But if nurses want to be heard, they will have to speak with their own authority, based on their own experience and their own values.

Finally, for sociology this book may remind us of what we should already know:

1. Morality is rooted in collective life. Since Durkheim, sociology has understood that moral beliefs are rooted in group membership and loyalty, and that such beliefs are arrived at neither through rational debate nor in isolation from other people. Durkheim also provided a model for the empirical study of morality, a topic too often left to philosophers and theologians.

2. What people say is not what people do. We should be cautious in using interviews to discover how people actually behave, since in interviews respondents report what they notice, whereas the unnoticed everyday routine may in fact be more important. The first of my three research projects for this book (in 1979) relied mainly on interviews; I switched my methods to first-hand observation after being disappointed with the misleading selective memories of several informants. In one interview, the head nurse on a pediatric research unit, an area in which any outsider would see tremendous ethical challenges, responded to my questions about ethics problems with repeated claims of "I just can't think of any." Without fieldwork to provide the meaning of her statement, it appears simply absurd.

3. Organizations are the dominant actors in our society. This book should reinforce the importance of organizations in our thinking about American society. To the layperson, this importance is not at all common wisdom; most Americans don't fully understand the power and pervasiveness of organizational, and especially corporate, influence.

4. Finally, subjective experience is not obvious. What "routinization" entails certainly is often not apparent to the nurses who live through it, nor is the objectification of patients always noted by hospital staff. The unexamined features of daily life are often the least noticed and possibly the most important features. And the scientific ethos of medicine (and of sociology) actually encourages the systematic rejection, as misleading, of the experience of our subjects. I think medicine's frequent cruelty comes from precisely this dismissal of the patients' experience as trivial or irrelevant. Sociology shouldn't make the same mistake, even if the consequences are less immediately felt.

A Final Note

Hospitals frighten me. Visiting them, I don't like their smell, I'm afraid other people will think I'm a patient, and I'm embarrassed by being healthy in the presence of sick people. At the same time, I don't *want* to be sick, much less be "a patient." I'm afraid of my vulnerability to disease, of which hospitals remind me; I'm afraid even of my own fear. Hospitals provoke all of this.

On the other hand, it's amazing what you can get used to. In this book, the reader, paralleling my own experience in doing the research, has seen many things, some shocking or grotesque. But these sights eventually have come to this end, and the reader probably has "gotten used to" the stories I have told. I certainly have. And as we become accustomed to the stories, we gradually start to accept them.

This is what happens to nurses and ironically, I think, it is the source of many of their problems. Nurses and their work reveal clearly to us how we overlook, ignore, and undervalue the crucial daily routines of which life (and death) are built. In nursing, the most important tasks are barely noticed; the most vital work is barely seen. Nurses are not central to the Big Events of the medical world. Official debates go on without them; policies are rendered without their thoughts or opinions being considered. Like women around the world who "only" gather and prepare food or give birth to and raise children, nurses are (predominantly) women who often do the most important work and get the least credit. While ethics committees debate abstract issues of principle in meeting rooms, nurses need bandages that stay on, soap that cleans without skin irritation, and enough staff to take care of the patients on the floor. Heart/lung machines are a fine thing, but nearly all patients would be happy to get some decent food. The realm of abstract arguments, high-technology research, and politically driven health care policies needs to acknowledge the realm of bedpans and beepers. The mundane must be respected.

So if we are to accomplish good in the world, I think it will be less through single, dramatic acts of moral courage than through relatively unglamorous, unnoticed lifetimes passed in (properly designed) organizational routines. When Florence

Nightingale stood up to the British army bureaucracy, she was inspiring, no doubt; those are the stories nurses sometimes share at their professional conferences. But she saved lives and comforted the dying by creating her own efficient, dedicated, fiercely disciplined nursing organization which as a matter of habit—of organizational culture—did the right things. People don't live only in bright visible moments of decision; they live, and die, and work in the ordinary everyday world. For sociologists and ethicists to understand and help people more, we should remember to live and work there, too.

Some readers may be interested in how I gathered the information reported in this book. The simple history of the research is unexceptional, but from talking with colleagues I gather that my success in gaining access to organizations and the trust of informants is notable and probably worth explaining.

The basic facts of the research, described in the opening sections of the book, are these: from January 1979 until June 1980 I worked in a large Northeastern medical center, mainly conducting interviews with some supporting observational studies. From June through August of 1982, I did some observations and a few interviews in a mid-sized (300 bed) community hospital also in the Northeast. From January until June of 1990, I did very intensive observational and interview research in a large medical center in the Southwest. The data used here include 110 formal interviews, 80 of them tape recorded, and my own on-site observations as recorded in several large boxes worth of field notes. In the text of this book, "Interview" signifies that the material is taken from a verbatim report of what an interviewee said; "Field Notes" indicates use of my contemporaneous account of events I personally witnessed.

Over the past fifteen years I have also visited, for short periods, many other hospitals and have spoken with countless nurses at conferences, social events, and in chance meetings of all kinds. In addition, I have read numerous books, magazines, and journal articles on nursing not formally cited in the notes.

This process, as I have said, is unexceptional. But the techniques I use for gaining access to settings and the trust of informants seem to be unusually successful. I share my own methods here for whatever benefit my professional colleagues may find in them.

"SIDE-IN ACCESS"

At a recent sociology convention, I attended a roundtable discussion by a dozen or so fellow sociologists who did research in hospitals. Early in the discussion someone commented on the difficulty in obtaining access to health care settings. Most people at the table instantly chimed in. A series of stories poured out, the point of which was that it was very difficult for sociologists to get permission to study hospitals, doctors, or indeed any medical settings. One speaker reported with no apparent embarrassment that her research proposals were rejected by five hospitals in a row; at a sixth, when the administrator turned her down, she (the sociologist) vented her frustration and berated the administrator for his ignorance, his hindering of science, and for his "lack of professionalism." Colleagues at the roundtable nodded approvingly. I understood why she was turned down.

I have never, either in this research or in that for an earlier book on Olympic-level competitive swimming,[1] been denied access to a targeted research setting. I call my standard approach "side-in" (as opposed to "top-down") access. This means that instead of seeking formal approval, at the outset, from an official administrator in charge, I use an informal series of contacts with lower level members of the organization. In the present study, I would try first to meet some staff nurses who worked at the target hospitals, see them socially—for instance, by inviting them to lunch—and tell them I was interested in learning about nursing, hospitals, and ethical problems therein. This gave me a chance, first, to learn a lot about nursing in a comfortable setting. More important, it gave the people I met a chance to see that I was easy to talk to, trustworthy, and a decent human being who was not out to do an exposé.

1. Daniel F. Chambliss, *Champions: The Making of Olympic Swimmers* (New York: William Morrow & Co., 1988).

Typically, such conversations ended with my new acquaintance suggesting that I talk with still another nurse or administrator and providing a phone number. I would immediately follow up on this suggestion. A series of such meetings and introductions typically concluded in my being invited by suitably authorized administrators to visit the hospital, observe various units, and talk with whomever I pleased. At that point, as needed, I would present a formal proposal for research, get necessary permission, and so on. Basically, my assumption is that once potential subjects get to know me, they won't be afraid of my doing research on them. This is the same technique I used in my research on Olympic swimming as well. It follows a guideline suggested to me in 1982 by Professor David Gray of Hamilton College, who said when I worried about getting access to difficult sites, "Ideally, they'll ask you to study them." Essentially, I never request access until I already know they'll say yes.

The "side-in" approach also recognizes that *official* access does not equal *real* access. In the smaller hospital I studied in 1982, a director of medical nursing, trying to be helpful, took me in tow on my first day in the hospital and dragged me around to meet every head nurse under her authority. It took me months to recover my credibility with those head nurses, who naturally enough saw me as somehow their boss's protégé or friend. In all settings, I have tried to maintain some visible distance from higher-ups, never calling them by first name or being seen with them in public, if possible.

The "side-in" approach has nearly produced failure for me only once. In the early months of my doctoral dissertation research in 1979, I had talked informally outside the hospital with three or four head nurses in the medical-surgical department of Northern General Hospital. I had already gotten well into research in several other departments of the hospital at this point and had received the approval of a variety of high administrators, including the director of nursing for the entire hospital. I then scheduled a meeting with the associate director for medical-surgical nursing to gain her approval to spend time in the units under her authority; I considered it a pro forma exercise at this point.

She didn't. When she realized that I had already talked

with a number of her people—albeit not in the hospital but on their own time—she became furious and demanded an explanation. I saw my dissertation research, well under way, about to go up in flames, and I realized that this woman held my professional fate in her hands. Worse, I had inadvertently violated her code, at least, of professional conduct. So I threw myself on her mercy: no excuses; I hadn't realized the mistake. I immediately offered, on the spot, to cease my *entire* thesis research project that instant, never use any of the material I had collected, abandon the topic itself, and start a new thesis project. I told her I had no idea that I had been doing anything wrong and had no intention at all of interfering either with her relations with her subordinates or with any of them doing their proper work. Basically, I (metaphorically) fell on the ground, begged forgiveness, and offered my bare neck to her sword.

Twenty minutes later I left her office with a kindly pat on the back and a list of names, offices, and phone numbers of all her subordinate managers and head nurses. She wanted to help in any way she could.

"DON'T WEAR A LAB COAT"

When I first began work at Northern General Hospital, a number of nurses asked me if I wanted to wear a white lab coat so as to "blend in" more with the hospital staff. When I asked my thesis adviser, Kai Erikson, if this was wise, he said (more or less), "Why would you wear a lab coat?" ("Uh . . . to look like a doctor.") "Are you a doctor? Just look like what you are, a graduate student doing thesis research. Don't wear a lab coat and don't shave off your beard either."

As usual, Erikson was right. You should look like who you are. Your appearance and behavior should convey that your motives are good and that you can be trusted to represent yourself honestly. In effect, wearing a lab coat or even passing oneself off as a "Doctor" tells those who know that one is willing to bend the truth or deceive people in getting access. And then they, rightly, assume that one would do the same with them. The minor short term disadvantages of being an odd figure (a social scientist) in the hospital are easily offset by the advantages of being genuinely trusted by one's informants.

EMPLOY "LAYERS OF CONFIDENTIALITY"

To gain the trust of informants you need to make your commitment to confidentiality obvious. One way to do this is to use what I call "layers of confidentiality," keeping information several layers deeper in confidence than is immediately required. Maintaining confidentiality of one's sources is a form of, basically, counterespionage, in which one's "opponents"—the curious—will try to put together pieces of information into an identifiable pattern. The best response is to "bury" confidential information behind multiple layers.

For instance: a key piece of confidential information in this book is who said what, that is, what real people made which statements, or were involved in which actions recorded here. I protect this information by (1) not identifying the hospitals studied to anyone not themselves a subject in the research; (2) studying multiple hospitals, so that no events can be clearly identified as occurring in any particular one; (3) not identifying any individuals by name; and (4) not confirming, even to other nurses in the same hospital or same unit, who I had interviewed. Occasionally this technique has assumed almost comic dimensions, as when I spoke individually with a cluster of friends who were nurses. They talked among themselves about the interviews, and I would continue to "neither affirm nor deny" that I had actually spoken with any of them. I did this with superiors who asked if I had interviewed subordinates. Not only, that is, did I not report who said what; I didn't report with whom I had spoken, or where. And I made this strategy public when asked. I believe that people talked freely with me in part because I was so public in refusing to share information, even with my own close informants.

In addition, I destroyed notes relating to legally problematic events, and all interview transcriptions that I didn't make myself were made by a small-town legal secretary who lives (no exaggeration) more than 1,000 miles from any of the research sites.

In the end, of course, none of this is still really sufficient.

OBSERVATION, NOT INTERVIEWS

Finally, I began the research relying heavily on tape-recorded interviews. These produced many dramatic stories and often confirmed theories I already held, but as I began to spend more time in hospitals I began to doubt the veracity of interviews. I began to see how the interviews were a reflection of my interests as much as of my subjects' lives. The stories told were more exciting than the ordinary drudgery I saw; the nurses described in stories seemed more committed and courageous than some of those I actually watched. Interviewees told what they noticed and remembered, which I discovered to be a highly selective version of what actually occurred. Much of life, I found, consists precisely in not noticing what one does all the time. "There aren't any ethical problems here I can think of," said a pediatric research nurse mentioned earlier; "You should talk with people on the ethics committee," said nurses gathered outside the room of an AIDS patient.

So interviews have provided telling quotations in this book and give support for some general points, but my major findings are based on firsthand observation.

In sum, the best attitude for carrying out effective fieldwork is simply to genuinely want to learn. This will encourage you to get close to your subjects, not to their bosses; to spend lots of time with people rather than rushing back to the comfort of your own office; to present yourself honestly, as who you are rather than as who you might like to be; to listen and watch, not talk and interfere; and to keep confidences rather than share gossip. It takes some self-discipline but rather minimal intelligence. All in all, high-quality fieldwork makes a nice example of what I've elsewhere called "the mundanity of excellence,"[2] the idea that excellence is less a matter of talent or extraordinary inborn ability and more likely the result of consistent, conscientious application of some basic, knowable techniques. Of course, quality fieldwork is also simply a wonderful way to meet interesting people and to learn about their lives.

2. Daniel F. Chambliss, "The Mundanity of Excellence: An Ethnographic Report on Stratification and Olympic Athletes," *Sociological Theory* (Spring 1989).